# Childbirth:

## Preparing for the Miracle

Marika Lee Connole
Phoenix, Arizona

ISBN 978-1-4357-2427-3

Published by Lulu.com

# Table of Contents

## Foreword

    I never thought I would write a book about childbirth. I didn't plan on doing it. But, through the years, I heard so many new mothers sharing awful stories of birth. So many women have had horrible birth experiences. Many have had just plain uninspiring birthing experiences. Nearly every woman I have talked to has a negative outlook about the birthing process. Because of this, I wished that they had discovered some things that I had discovered along the way. I have had numerous people ask me how I can stand to have babies without medical intervention in the form of drugs. I have also had people tell me how I am so "brave" to have had most of my children at home. I am neither extremely pain tolerant nor particularly brave. So, that is where this book came into being. I offer a very simple outlook on how your body works during labor and delivery, advice that really works on what to do mentally to prepare beforehand and during labor, and how to make the overall birth experience a spiritual one. Included in the book are personal accounts of the births of each of my children.

www.completelee.com

## Preface

The most glorious event ever to take place on this earth was a birth. It was the birth of a Savior, Jesus Christ. His birth was foretold by prophets many years prior to the event. Signs and wonders surrounded His birth. Angels by the multitudes rejoiced in the heavens because of Christ's birth. It is still talked about today. There is a season of the year that is devoted exclusively to celebrate His birth. His birth happened on a sacred, silent, holy night. It was a miracle.

Today, every time a newborn babe enters the world, it is reminiscent of that Christ child. There is nothing more wondrous than holding a baby that has just left the hands of God and feeling the love that emanates from that precious child. Knowing this, why should we not prepare to have a great spiritual experience for the birth of a child? Every birth has the potential to be a great spiritually uplifting experience.

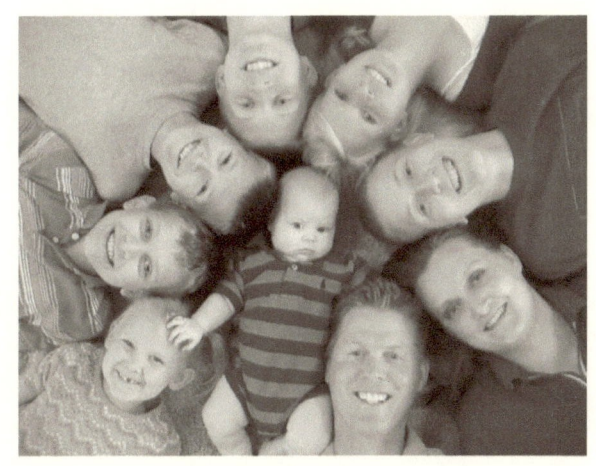

Our Family Circle

Chapter I—What is this book all about?

This is a spiritual book. Birth is a spiritual thing. Nowhere is God's love more evident than in a newborn babe. Our Father in Heaven knew what he was doing when he created us. Satan, the Father of Lies, wants us to believe the widespread notion about birth that displays birth as a horrid, painful experience that we must endure in martyr-like fashion. Trying to think in terms of hard work, concentration and spirituality in the miracle of birth is to be the focus of this book. Birth, the taking part in a new life coming to earth, is a wondrous and beautiful event.

Before we came to this earth, we lived in a wonderful place. We were well acquainted with our Heavenly Father and Jesus Christ. I can hardly imagine how loved we must have felt. We trusted in Him. We knew He had a perfect plan. We were excited about the opportunity to love and serve Him when our chance came to come to earth. I think we were full of hope while basking in His glorious presence.

Your sweet baby that is about to come to you has just left that majestic place to now make his home with you. He is very excited to see what earth has to offer. He is radiant with love, particularly for you, his parents, for allowing him to join your wonderful family. I imagine he hopes that you will make many preparations to make his initial glimpse of life a joyous, spiritual experience. Having just come from the presence of God, this little one could experience an awful trauma if his arrival is not met with loving arms, kind words and a beautiful atmosphere. He will have a more smooth transition if his parents have invited his friends, the angels, to help in his birth. Pray for the Spirit of God to be in the room as you welcome your new baby, the child sent by God to you.

What can you do to prepare for a wonderful, spiritual, uplifting birth experience? Most of us know that a new baby comes straight from God. I believe that God can help prepare you for your new little miracle better than anyone else.

It is my intention to offer some suggestions which have helped me in many aspects of the pregnancy and births of my 7 children. I would like to share with you what I have learned, through my experiences, about physical health, mental preparation and spiritual preparation for birth.

In no way do I think that I have all the answers. I know that there are many circumstances that I haven't even thought of or experienced. But, I do know that Heavenly Father hears and answers prayers. I believe that He will allow anyone who seeks to do so to have a spiritual experience at birth. It doesn't matter whether that experience takes place in the hospital, at home, or some other location, or whether there is a cesarean delivery, breech, or "normal" birth.

I know each person has to find her own way to do things. If someone needs specific help, kneel in prayer and ask the One who is sure to help. I am hoping that by sharing my experiences that I can help others find, with God's help, the best way for their family. Certainly everyone won't want to do things the same way I do, nor do I expect it. I simply am giving these things as ideas for others to consider. Hopefully those who read these words will find some truths they can use.

Chapter II—Taking care of you

One of the first things you can do to prepare for the birth of your precious baby is to allow yourself to take care of you. This is true, even <u>before</u> conceiving!  If mommy is in good condition, baby will have a better time trying to make it to earth. Ask Heavenly Father to help you be strong in resisting unhealthy foods.  I often would ask myself questions, such as, "Is this what you would like your pure new baby to be eating?" and "Can you eat good things for your baby if you don't want to do it for yourself sometimes?"  Or "What would Heavenly Father think would be best for my baby?"  Talking to yourself will often help. Tell your baby that you are trying to do the best you can for him. He will appreciate that.  Try to make nutritious & protein-rich snacks to be readily available for you.  Some things I think are good include:

- Apple slices with peanut butter
- Celery sticks kept in the fridge in water, already washed
- Carrot sticks kept in the fridge in water, already washed
- Granola by the handful (Homemade is best of course! ☺)
- Nuts & seeds
- Raisins
- A glass of milk with 1 Tbs blackstrap molasses (great iron source)
- Leftover brown rice with a dab of butter and dill
- Fruits

- Veggies
- Protein shakes, especially with add-ins
- Juice popsicles

I am providing a bunch of easy recipes for snacks and some meals at the back of the book, so be sure to check there too.

Eat things God has provided on the earth for you. Try to steer clear of processed and refined foods. Be sure to do the best YOU can. If you really try to give your baby the best you feel you can, you have no reason to let yourself feel guilty if you don't "do better". God will bless you for the efforts you make. If you splurge, do not be mad at yourself. You do the best you can for your baby. Don't overburden yourself by trying to be perfect all at once!

## Section 2

Another way to make sure you are at your best physically is to get the rest you need. This can be difficult, especially if you have other children! If you don't feel you have gotten enough rest at night, you can at least allow yourself to relax, sit down for a few minutes now and then. Even though it is hard to talk yourself into believing it, a rest for you is far more important than getting the dishes or other housework done.

Section 3

Husbands, you can be involved in the preparation for your new one. Isn't it nice to know there are some things you can do to help your sweet new baby to have a pleasant arrival into this world? Here are some ideas.

Compliment your wife when you see her trying to do her best.

Allow your wife to take a nap if she needs it and you are home. Just think, sometimes a nap means the difference between a cranky wife and a happy one or the difference between dinner on the table vs. peanut butter sandwiches!

You know your wife will be hungry often. Bring her some healthy food to snack on. Encourage her to eat good things. After all, this is your baby she is feeding. Eat good things with her.

As the birth of our second child approached, I told my husband that I would take responsibility for the newborn at night and he could have responsibility for our first child. This is actually quite a good deal for husbands. Instead of getting up every two to three hours throughout the night every night to nurse a baby, you only have to get up on occasion, sometimes being allowed the blessing of an entire complete night of sleep! This deal is extremely helpful to Mom, especially when you have many small children as we did. We were able to get to the point where we trained ourselves to hear only specific children. Kevin was always very good about getting up with the other kids. I appreciated this so much. It is a sacrifice to lose some of your sleep to get up with a child at night, but it is helping your wife with the birth of your next child too.

Section 4

One more thing for your physical well-being is to try to get some exercise. I don't mean going for a strenuous run, doing jumping jacks, lifting weights. Simple things, like going for a walk on a sunny day and breathing in good fresh air. This will help you clear your mind and get your muscles moving too. Just keep yourself active to promote overall well-being.

Section 5

In addition to eating well, getting sufficient rest and exercise, I feel that vitamin and herb supplements can play an important role in your health and delivery. I am not a doctor or an herbalist, but these are a few things that I have learned and that I feel have helped me.

Vitamin C helps to make a stretchy and strong bag of waters. If the bag is not strong, you have the potential of it breaking prematurely. Vitamin C is also good for keeping your energy level up. Emergen-C packets from Alacer are one of my favorite ways to take vitamin C. You just pour the powder into your favorite juice. It tastes good and picks you up a bit.

About 800-1200 IU of natural vitamin E per day, especially in the last trimester can aid you with getting enough oxygen during labor. This of course means that your baby will get what he needs as well. He will be a nice healthy color.

Calcium (I liked the liquid kind with magnesium) can help keep you from getting cramps (Charlie horses) in the calf of your leg. If you do get a cramp, you can alleviate the pain almost instantly by pulling your foot towards your shin and holding it there. Not always easy to do when you become very round, but someone else can do it for you if need be. I didn't get these too often, but when they did occur, it was usually at night for me, so Kevin could help if I needed it.

A good natural prenatal multiple vitamin is also a good idea for getting yourself overall nutrients. I guess you can view this as a little insurance policy for getting what you need.

Iron is the other supplement I wanted to mention. A natural form of iron can help prevent you from getting anemia and keep your energy level up. Black strap molasses is excellent for this, as is red raspberry leaf tea. Iron that is not natural can actual make you feel sick.

God intended for us to use the herbs he provided for us. Psalms 104:14 tells us herbs are for the service of man.

"He causeth the grass to grow for the cattle, and herb for the service of man: that he may bring forth food out of the earth;"

Doctrine & Covenants 59:17-20 reads:

17 Yea, and the herb, and the good things which come of the earth, whether for food or for raiment, or for houses, or for barns, or for orchards, or for gardens, or for vineyards;

18 Yea, all things which come of the earth, in the season thereof, are made for the benefit and the use of man, both to please the eye and to gladden the heart;

19 Yea, for food and for raiment, for taste and for smell, to strengthen the body and to enliven the soul.

20 And it pleaseth God that he hath given all these things unto man; for unto this end were they made to be used, with judgment, not to excess, neither by extortion.

Herbs, unlike drugs, are generally safe to take when you are pregnant. Herbs should be used with good judgment. It is always good to consult someone who has studied much about them if you are planning to use them. You can also learn a lot about herbs by studying good books yourself.

If you are taking some drugs as prescribed by your doctor, it would be a good idea to let him know what herbs or other supplements you are taking as well.

The best all-around pregnancy herb is red raspberry leaf. It strengthens the uterus and the female organs. It is soothing if you feel worn out. It is tasty with just a bit of honey. I tried to drink at least a cup per day. You can also take the capsules if you wanted. After giving birth in three years in a row, my uterus still did its job well on the third child and is still in good condition. I attribute a lot of that to the red raspberry leaf tea.

A few other herbs I have found useful include cayenne, blue cohosh, and St. Johnswort. Cayenne capsules help stop bleeding. Blue cohosh can help keep labor progressing and St. Johnswort is good for afterpains. Study up on these herbs in order to learn more for yourself.

As a little side note, an herbal combination called Femmend from Nature's Way is a good herb to take if you are trying to conceive. I know many women who have been able to conceive after strengthening their female organs with this product. (Again, this is a pre-pregnancy herbal combination)

## Chapter III—Inviting the Spirit of God

Let's start on a clean slate. Erase from your mind all thoughts of birth experiences you have heard of or been through yourself. Easier said than done, I know.

Now, pretend you are the first woman on earth—Eve. I suppose that Eve was a very healthy woman. I imagine she took good care of herself, eating all those good fruits in the garden and later tilling the earth alongside Adam. She was the first woman to give birth. What do you suppose she thought? She knew absolutely nothing about having a baby. I imagine she must have wondered about it. Facing the unknown can be intimidating. Where did she turn for help?

Eve knew her Father in Heaven's plan was a good one. Therefore, she knew she could trust in Him. It was to Him she turned for help in this uncertain time, I am sure. If she had any worries, the Lord would encourage her. God would provide her with information as needed. In fact, He could guide her through her pregnancy, labor and delivery.

One way that Eve was blessed was in the fact that she had no one telling her of negative experiences they had had. Consequently, she could create her own experience. Eve wanted children. She knew that was part of Heavenly Father's plan for her. Since she trusted in her Heavenly Father, how could she not believe that He would allow her to have a good, positive, spiritual experience where God and his angels would help her?

The same is true for each woman who seeks. The Lord will uphold you spiritually, physically and emotionally. He loves you and wants you to have good experiences. With a loving Father and his angels ushering your new babe to earth, how can we help but believe it will be a grand event?

We are blessed today because we have seen a new baby. They radiate God's love. They have skin softer than silk. They make the sweetest noises the human ear has ever heard. What can compare to holding a precious, newly bathed baby up next to your check and inhaling deeply? They smell so good. These little beings have just come straight from the presence of God. Eve had never seen a baby or touched that soft skin, but I would imagine that her heart must have been full of anticipation.

Eve trusted that Heavenly Father knew what He was doing when He designed the human body. He's the master that created everything and his greatest creation was and still is the human being.

As we go along, try to imagine to yourself what a loving Father in Heaven would want for you.

Prayer is powerful. Here are some prayer ideas for pregnancy and birth.

- Prayerfully inviting children to come to join your lives can bless and enrich a life more than anything.
- Earnestly petitioning the Lord on behalf of your unborn child strengthens faith.

- Praying for a husband to know the things to say and do as he becomes a coach, a comforter, and a support before he becomes a father.
- Husband praying for a wife to be able to feel strong, in control and able to feel the spirit of angels present with her at birth.
- Praying together for each other and the baby.
- Praying that your baby will be able to have a smooth, safe journey and be able to feel your love once he gets here.
- Pray for your doctor or midwife to be able to know your needs, as well as your baby's needs and to help you have a special experience.

## Section 2

Ask Heavenly Father to help you find a doctor or midwife that will allow you to have the kind of experience the Lord would want for you to have. The person "in charge" at the time of delivery has a great deal to do with the tone or mood present at your baby's birth. A doctor or midwife has a great responsibility resting on his or her shoulders. I believe a doctor or midwife should be a very Christ-like person. Someone who brings precious new spirits from heaven into this world needs to be a man or woman of God. If they are in tune with the Spirit of the Lord, He can inspire them to know what to do if a life needs to be saved, or if damage to a mother or child can be avoided.

Consider these words from Brigham Young: "Who is the real doctor? That man who knows by the spirit of revelation what ails an individual and by the same spirit knows what medicine to administer." (Brigham Young Journal of Discourses 15:226)

That gave me some food for thought.

It is sad that so many babies today are born into the hands of a person who has forgotten, or has never accepted, God. After delivering hundreds of babies, it could be easy to take for granted the miracle. Finding someone who still reveres this sacred event really helps to bring the Spirit into the room. Finding a doctor or midwife that really cares about people, really cares about what they are doing is very important. It is nice to feel like a person instead of "just another number". Take the time to choose even before you are expecting, if you can.

With my first child, I didn't "shop around" at all for a doctor. I went with the doctor my insurance plan placed me with. While there was nothing completely horrid about this man, I never got a sense that he cared about me or my child as patients. I always felt he probably spouted off the same exact comments to every woman he dealt with. When the time came for labor and delivery, he wasn't at all concerned with what I had in mind for the birth of my baby. He definitely tried to get me to do things his way and was in an obvious hurry to be done with me as quickly as possible. He got visibly irritated with Kevin and me when we didn't want certain medical procedures done. By the time the baby had arrived, he was actually rather angry.

I include that last paragraph simply because I know that it was very nice with the births of my other children, not to have to deal with an unyielding doctor. You have to remember that you and your husband are the ones that are in charge of the birth. You are paying the doctor or midwife for their assistance and expertise, which is a much needed and valued thing. But a doctor or midwife does not have the right to play ruthless dictator in the event or to bring in a negative spirit. Neither of those things helps with the birth.

Section 3

Your baby is coming to earth after having been surrounded by people who love him. As the baby is growing and developing inside you, allow a little bit of heaven into your home. The baby is under stress when mother is. Taking time for personal scripture study and prayer will make you feel happier. It will be better for the baby as well.

Having the Spirit of the Lord reside in your home provides a ready environment for your baby to come to. Whether the birth takes place at home, or in a hospital, you can take that Spirit with you. While 5 out of 7 of my children were born at home, and I like that atmosphere for birth, I have come to realize that the Lord can be with you wherever you are. You just have to bring a little bit of home with you.

## Section 4

Satan, the Devil, the Father of Lies, does not want children to be born. And if they are born, he wouldn't prefer for them to be born into homes where there is a married, loving mother and father waiting.

Satan promotes that which is sacred as something commonplace. He encourages sexual promiscuity and then advocates being irresponsible. So many babies are born to unwed, often teenage, mothers. Statistics are astonishing. Sadly, many millions of babies are being aborted each year. How God must weep over this.

Satan has many ideas to thwart our Heavenly Father's plan. When he can't stop a baby from coming, he will attempt to make birth an awful experience. Satan has his hand in Hollywood. Nearly every movie made (actually I would say every movie that I have ever seen) that includes a birth, shows a screaming, terrified mother who is in so much pain that she must have drugs administered before, during and after the birth. The exception would be pioneer type movies in which the mother either dies a tragic death, or endures excruciating pain and torment.

It is not a wonder to me why so many mothers do not look forward to giving birth. This definitely does not need to be the case. I sincerely believe that by inviting the Lord to help you throughout pregnancy and delivery, you do not need to fear the birth experience. You can look forward to it with knowledge and even excitement knowing that God and his angels are there to help you.

Don't get me wrong, giving birth is extremely hard work! (Thus the term labor) I have chosen to think in terms of hard work and concentration instead of thinking in terms of fear and pain. Am I saying I have never experienced either of those things in a birth? No. But I am saying that I know when my mind is focused on what I have been training it to focus on, then my mind thinks of dwelling on concentrating on the task at hand – that of working with and not against my body. It is when I have a lapse in my mind or allow fear that I feel pain in such a way that I feel I can't continue. If I refocus my mind on what it needs to focus on, then I have somewhat of a buffer from pain. The process of giving birth is certainly not a challenge you would want to tackle on a daily basis. But it is wonderful to know you can receive strength and courage when you need it. And to know you can work with your body, rather than against it to help things along makes you feel like you are really doing something to help your baby get to you.

When the baby comes and is laid in your arms, you are filled with thankfulness, incredible thankfulness, vitality, and energy just from the thought of this miracle and the immense love you feel for those around you. A natural feeling of euphoria envelops you.

In today's society, we, unlike Eve, are subject to pollutions of food, air, water, media corruption and the like. But, we can rejoice in knowing that the God she called upon will be available to us as He was to her. A truly sobering thought.

Chapter IV—How your body works

I have learned a few things along the way that have proven useful in child bearing. Before and after the birth of my first child I studied many books to learn about birth and about how the body works. It really is an amazing thing. God prepared woman's body to naturally give birth to a child. Working with the body's natural abilities, makes labor and delivery a better experience.

Even before you go in to labor, your body automatically does things to prepare. One of these things is that your hips widen. Also, your bones soften. The perineal area is made to stretch wide. The muscles there are very elastic. All of these things the Lord put in place so that the process of birth can happen.

Here is a simple diagram of what is on the inside, so you have that for easy reference.

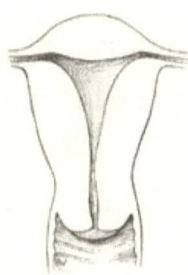

When the baby is ready to come, the pituitary gland releases oxytocin, which causes the uterus to start contracting. A contracting muscle is simply a muscle that is working as it should, tightening and releasing. This is what happens at the beginning of labor. The uterine muscles begin tightening and then relaxing, tightening and then relaxing.

A typical scenario would begin with contractions that start in kind of a warm-up stage. They start off small and relatively far apart. As things continue, they get progressively stronger and closer together.

When the uterine muscles tighten, they cause the cervix to widen and flatten. This is what is meant by dilate and efface. This is to prepare your baby to be able to enter the birth canal and be born.

## Section 2

Let's take a closer look at things. Your body naturally produces the hormone oxytocin. The physician's replacement for this is called pitocin.

Pitocin is commonly given to artificially start (induce) a woman in to labor. This is often done for convenience sake or when the doctor has determined that the baby is ready or thinks it would be harmful for the baby to remain in utero.

Anyone can look up pitocin in the Physician's Desk Reference (PDR). Pitocin is said to control postpartum hemorrhage, but one of the adverse reactions to the drug, listed in the PDR, is actually postpartum hemorrhage. This doesn't make too much sense to my mind. This, as well as other possible adverse reactions and the very, very precise instructions for use, make me very leery of this product.

As a rule, a baby is best off coming when he says he is ready. Then the body's natural hormones will help him come. If an artificial hormone is used to start contractions, a little too much for one person may not be enough for another person. If a mother gets too much of the hormone, she may have very strong contractions right away and consequently not be able to stay in control of her birth experience to any degree. The oxytocin that comes from the pituitary gland delivers the exact right dosage for that particular woman. Sounds like God's handiwork again.

Most babies will come when they are ready. If you feel, for some reason or another, that your baby is actually "overdue", ask your Heavenly Father about what to do. Perhaps asking for help that your baby will be ready to come and that your body will perform as needed at the exact right time is all that it will take to do the trick. Predicting the exact date of birth is not a perfected science, particularly if unsure of the date of the mother's last period. Dates can be wrong. Don't put all your hopes in them. Having had babies come "early" and "late" and close to on time, I know it is hard not to hope for THE day not to go past!

Pitocin is often used after a baby's birth as well to control hemorrhaging. I was told by my first doctor that every mother had to have a shot of pitocin after delivery or suffer severe hemorrhaging, possibly even to the point of bleeding to death. I was also told that if he did not give it, my doctor could have a malpractice suit on his hands. Even with his strict warning, my choice was to not take the drug. And, in case you are wondering, I did not sue him, nor did I bleed to death.

Here I must pause to say that if a mother is losing blood fast, having pitocin would be a better choice than having to get a blood transfusion or worse. A drug can be a lot faster-acting than an herb, particularly when they can inject it directly into your bloodstream. Trying to use herbal remedies, or keeping an eye on the blood flow before just automatically administering a shot of pitocin, would be my preferred method. But, if the bleeding is not getting under control, the mother's health is in danger. At this time, under good judgment, pitocin would be more of a benefit than a harm. There is a place for drugs; I just don't feel they should be commonplace. As a general rule, natural is best.

## Section 3

When your uterus starts to contract, this is an exciting time! As a first time mother, I had no idea what a contraction felt like. I had actually thought I would get sharp pains in the area of the birth canal. I was of course, very wrong. Somehow I didn't find a good explanation of what to expect in a contraction with all my studying.

Sometimes early labor can be confusing. I have to admit that even with seven kids, I wasn't always right when I thought I was going in to labor. With my first child I wound up figuring out quite quickly that labor was happening, simply because my body was doing something it had never done before. Things happened pretty much the same way with my second child, so I was able to realize I was in labor then. Child number three I had thought I was in labor on one occasion only to find out it was false labor. Child four threw me for a loop several times. With child number five I had sent my midwife home only to have her come back a few hours later. Finally with child number six, things proceeded about the same way they did with child number one! I thought it was pretty ridiculous not to be able to tell when I was in labor with consecutive children, but I've been told that this is actually a common occurrence.

So, what does a contraction feel like? You can feel as well as see when a contraction is happening. If you look at your belly, you can actually see it becoming very hard over all. You can also feel the muscles in your tummy tightening.

At first it isn't very bothersome. Often with early contractions, you can read, crochet, write, walk around or whatever you feel like doing. It wouldn't be good to do anything physically straining because your uterus is already beginning to "work-out" and you have physical work (labor) coming up that you will need your strength for. Your body will be tired when you are through.

One way to tell if you are experiencing real labor is to try and feel if the contraction is all the way in the inner core of the muscles. If not, it may be just Braxton-Hicks contractions. Braxton-Hicks contractions can occur in the final trimester and are what could be called "practice" contractions. I didn't experience these at all with my first two children. With number seven, they were a regularly occurring nuisance. Braxton-Hicks can become rhythmic; leading you to believe that it might be the real thing. A good doctor or midwife will never make you feel dumb for thinking you are in labor when you actually aren't. My midwife told me that about 75% of women that head to the hospital are sent home because of false labor. So, if it happens to you, you are not alone!

One of the best things to do when you go into labor is to have a priesthood blessing. Having your husband pray for you and the baby is such a comforting and reassuring thing.

Section 4

As labor progresses, be sure to keep positive and happy thoughts in your mind. Be completely and thoroughly relaxed. You can focus on your new little miracle. Or, focus on the act of relaxing itself.

If you have any trouble keeping calm and in control, ask Heavenly Father to help you find something to gain and keep control. Some people like to breathe certain ways; others stare at a certain object during a contraction. Still others like to be talked to or coached through it. With some of my births I chose to watch the clock. That way I would know approximately how long the contraction would last. If my contractions were one minute long, then I would feel good about things when the clock made it to the 30 second mark. Sometimes when it seems hard to be in control for the full minute, it helps to break that down into smaller segments. Another idea is to visualize a serene scene. Sometimes a combination of things is what is needed.

Through each pregnancy, I kept studying and trying to find things that worked better than the time before. My best labors started with baby number five. What I chose to do is to visualize during contractions. I didn't visualize a serene scene. I visualized what my body was doing on the inside and how I was allowing my mind to help facilitate what my body was naturally trying to do. There will be more on visualization in an upcoming chapter.

As delivery time approaches, a mom needs the most support. An inspired coach can really help. Praise and encouragement are often just what is needed. Recognizing that the baby is that much closer to being here with you is a great reminder. Angels in attendance can be a comforting thought. Affirming that mom is so strong, brave and in control can be helpful. Again, a good coach will have to watch to see what the new mom needs. It can be different things, even for the same mom. So, fathers, watch and pray to be inspired!

Section 5

After the cervix has dilated and effaced completely, the baby is free to move into the birth canal. Your baby is nearly here!

This is the point at which an urge to push may be felt. You won't want to be laying flat on your back. You will want gravity to be able to do some of the work!

It is important at this point to be sure to work with what your body is doing. Visualizing is very helpful. Being able to sense what is happening inside yourself will help your mind encourage the natural flow of things. Pay attention to what you are feeling and then do what you feel you should to allow things to progress smoothly. If you push too aggressively at the wrong times, you may tear. The doctor or midwife should let you know if they see anything to suggest you should slow down. Once the baby has crowned, it is not a good idea to push.

Relaxation is a powerful tool throughout labor and delivery. I will explain this more thoroughly later as well as offer ideas on how to do it. Allow yourself to relax and work with your body and not against. If you are fearful of birth and resist against what your body is naturally designed to do, your muscles will be tense. If you are tense, your muscles will be hard and tight. Your baby will come more smoothly and easily when your muscles are relaxed, which allows the muscles to stretch. Your body is designed with a lot of elasticity to allow that baby to come out. If your muscles are tight, chances are great that you will tear, even badly. Or, there is the alternative called an episiotomy.

An episiotomy is a surgical procedure. The doctor will cut you so that you don't tear. Most doctors routinely give episiotomies, especially for the birth of the first child. The doctor I had with my first child told me that I would tear severely (to put it mildly) if I didn't have one. He also told me it is easier to mend a straight cut than a jagged cut. I believe it is easier for doctor to sew a straight cut, but I believe it is easier for a body to mend a jagged cut.

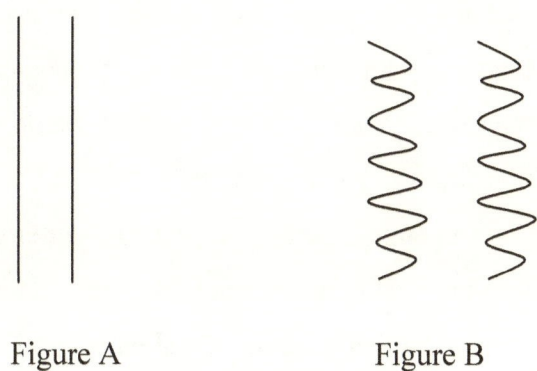

Figure A                    Figure B

A doctor can quickly sew a straight cut, as shown in figure A. The body has a harder time mending a straight cut. If you have ever had a paper cut, you know this to be true. The body must suture it together in new places. Figure B shows how a tear naturally goes back together. It would be more difficult to sew, yes, but it goes back together like a jigsaw puzzle. This is easier for the body to hold together.

If you get an episiotomy, you will pay for that procedure as well as having the discomfort of being cut. The other bad news is that you might be getting cut unnecessarily! Nothing says you have to be cut or tear. You can have a baby without either tearing or being cut.

I have 3 suggestions to help avoid an episiotomy: relaxation, visualization and vitamin E oil. These things, in addition to letting your doctor know you don't want to have an episiotomy if at all possible.

As I stated earlier, relaxation can be a powerful tool. When your baby has started down the birth canal, you can't just call it quits. The baby will come. There's no turning back!

If you can keep your mind from tension, you can keep your body from tension. Your focus at this point should be on what your body is doing to get the baby here. Feel and sense everything that is happening. Allow your face to be relaxed. The face shows when you are not relaxed elsewhere. During contractions and pushing there should be tightening and stressing in the right way. The tightening and stressing that is not good, would be that which works against what the body is trying to do. In between contractions, your body should be relaxed but on the ready for the work it needs to do when another contraction comes. When a contraction comes, focus your energies into allowing your uterine muscles to work, while keeping the rest of your body relaxed.

If you can learn to relax, visualization should come easily to you as well, because they go hand in hand. Visualizing should be practiced during pregnancy, so that it is quickly called to mind during labor. What should you visualize? Here is one possible picture.

*I see myself ready to give birth to my new miracle baby. I am calm and in control. My mind is working in exact coordination with my body. I can see in my mind how the muscles and tissues in the vaginal area are very relaxed. I am willing the baby to come. With each contraction I push in complete accordance with my body's capacity. The muscles and tissues are actually stretching wider and wider to accommodate the baby. I push gently enough to make sure my muscles and tissues have enough time to continue stretching wide enough for the baby's head. As the baby's head is crowning, I cease pushing but focus on the perineal area widening enough to accommodate the baby's head. Next come the shoulders. My body stretches again to allow the shoulders through. After that the little body slides effortlessly out and I see my new little son or daughter.*

As you practice relaxing, you can visualize this scenario, or something similar adapted to your own words. If you visualize this over and over throughout your pregnancy, your mind will be at ease. If you are prepared, you won't be fearful. Fear causes tension and stress. Your mind will know exactly what is going to take place at the time of your baby's birth. It will then be able to relax and not be fearful. Your mind will not cause you to resist the birth. You will remember what you visualized when it is actually happening and then act accordingly.

The third thing you can do to help avoid an episiotomy is to do perineal massages. Use a good vitamin E oil. Start about 4 weeks or more before your due date. If you feel comfortable with it, your spouse can help you with this. Make sure you are relaxed. Rub oil onto clean fingers. Work the oil into your muscles and tissues as you stretch the area. Massage and stretch (gently pull) outwardly just until you feel a slight burning sensation. Then hold until the burning subsides. Repeat this procedure until you have done the whole perineal area. Do this each night if you can for about 5 minutes. After doing this for a few days, you will notice that your body has become more pliable, able to stretch a little further. When you notice more pliability, you can just massage every other day or so until the baby comes. Practice being relaxed with the rest of your body while the stretching is taking place. This is good practice for the real deal. This exercise is particularly good for first time mothers.

Remember that your hips widen, which provides more room for the baby. Also, your bones have softened to help if the baby needs to press against them. The baby's skull bones are very soft and can contour to the shape provided him if necessary. Heavenly Father provided for every detail necessary in birth. He didn't forget a thing.  He knows what your body needs to do to have a baby.

## Chapter V:  Preparing for Labor and Delivery

Labor. What is labor?  The word labor often means work, usually hard physical work.  Hard physical work usually means that when you are done you are perhaps weary; your muscles have been greatly exercised and may ache.

Labor, when it pertains to birth, is best thought of in these same terms.  Your uterine muscles will work and your mind will exercise as well.

Labor is hard work, but it shouldn't be excruciating pain. It is very hard work and it gets much harder the closer to the birth it gets.  Your muscles are contracting over and over again. They are very tired.  It is like running farther when you feel you can't run another step and you do anyway.  And your muscles cry at you to stop.  But you don't stop.  You keep going until you finally reach your destination.  Then, you slowly wind down.

After the baby is born, your body will be physically tired. If you have had a natural birth, complete with Divine help, you will feel rejuvenated and somewhat invigorated of mind even though your physical body is tired.  This is because of the wonderful spiritual experience, the miracle, you have just been a part of.

Knowing that labor is hard work, it is good to prepare your mind and body for the experience.  Let's take a look at this.

First of all, what can you do to get your mind "in shape"? The brain exercise called visualization is great.

There are numerous books written to extensively cover the subject of visualization. I will just explain the procedure I have used for the births of my children that has worked well for me. If you desire more information, check the library or bookstore.

Section 2

Seek inspiration from the Lord in your visualizing. If you are going to be part of a miracle, it makes sense to enlist the help of the Lord, the source of all miracles.

There is a scripture in James 1: 5 that tells us to seek the Lord's help when we need wisdom.

"If any of you lack wisdom, let him ask of God, that giveth to all men liberally, and upbraideth not; and it shall be given him. But let him ask in faith, nothing wavering."

Have you ever asked God for something and received it? Have you ever prayed doubtfully for something?

Christ taught us to ask and doubt not. There are quite a few scriptures that stress the importance of belief and of not doubting. Two of my favorites are Matthew 21:17-22 and Acts 10:17-19.

In Matthew, Jesus tells his disciples that they can do anything through faithful prayers without doubting.

17 ¶ And he left them, and went out of the city into Bethany; and he lodged there.

18 Now in the morning as he returned into the city, he hungered.

19 And when he saw a fig tree in the way, he came to it, and found nothing thereon, but leaves only, and said unto it, Let no fruit grow on thee henceforward for ever. And presently the fig tree withered away.

20 And when the disciples saw *it,* they marvelled, saying, How soon is the fig tree withered away!

21 Jesus answered and said unto them, Verily I say unto you, If ye have faith, and doubt not, ye shall not only do this *which is done* to the fig tree, but also if ye shall say unto this mountain, Be thou removed, and be thou cast into the sea; it shall be done.

22 And all things, whatsoever ye shall ask in prayer, believing, ye shall receive.


The scripture in Acts talks about Peter, an apostle. He was very human—he doubted.

17 Now while Peter doubted in himself what this vision which he had seen should mean, behold, the men which were sent from Cornelius had made enquiry for Simon's house, and stood before the gate,

18 And called, and asked whether Simon, which was surnamed Peter, were lodged there.

19 ¶ While Peter thought on the vision, the Spirit said unto him, Behold, three men seek thee.

We know that the Lord can do anything, but sometimes we doubt ourselves! We have to keep in mind that we are children of God. If he has inspired us to do something, we can do it.

Mormon 9:9-11, 15-21, 24-28 instructs us about living our lives so that we may be worthy of partaking in a miracle.

9 For do we not read that God is the same yesterday, today, and forever, and in him there is no variableness neither shadow of changing?

10 And now, if ye have imagined up unto yourselves a god who doth vary, and in whom there is shadow of changing, then have ye imagined up unto yourselves a god who is not a God of miracles.

11 But behold, I will show unto you a God of miracles, even the God of Abraham, and the God of Isaac, and the God of Jacob; and it is that same God who created the heavens and the earth, and all things that in them are.

15 And now, O all ye that have imagined up unto yourselves a god who can do no miracles, I would ask of you, have all these things passed, of which I have spoken? Has the end come yet? Behold I say unto you, Nay; and God has not ceased to be a God of miracles.

16 Behold, are not the things that God hath wrought marvelous in our eyes? Yea, and who can comprehend the marvelous works of God?

17 Who shall say that it was not a miracle that by his word the heaven and the earth should be; and by the power of his word man was created of the dust of the earth; and by the power of his word have miracles been wrought?

18 And who shall say that Jesus Christ did not do many mighty miracles? And there were many mighty miracles wrought by the hands of the apostles.

19 And if there were miracles wrought then, why has God ceased to be a God of miracles and yet be an unchangeable Being? And behold, I say unto you he changeth not; if so he would cease to be God; and he ceaseth not to be God, and is a God of miracles.

20 And the reason why he ceaseth to do miracles among the children of men is because that they dwindle in unbelief, and depart from the right way, and know not the God in whom they should trust.

21 Behold, I say unto you that whoso believeth in Christ, doubting nothing, whatsoever he shall ask the Father in the name of Christ it shall be granted him; and this promise is unto all, even unto the ends of the earth.

24 And these signs shall follow them that believe—in my name shall they cast out devils; they shall speak with

new tongues; they shall take up serpents; and if they drink any deadly thing it shall not hurt them; they shall lay hands on the sick and they shall recover;

25 And whosoever shall believe in my name, doubting nothing, unto him will I confirm all my words, even unto the ends of the earth.

26 And now, behold, who can stand against the works of the Lord? Who can deny his sayings? Who will rise up against the almighty power of the Lord? Who will despise the works of the Lord? Who will despise the children of Christ? Behold, all ye who are despisers of the works of the Lord, for ye shall wonder and perish.

27 O then despise not, and wonder not, but hearken unto the words of the Lord, and ask the Father in the name of Jesus for what things soever ye shall stand in need. Doubt not, but be believing, and begin as in times of old, and come unto the Lord with all your heart, and work out your own salvation with fear and trembling before him.

28 Be wise in the days of your probation; strip yourselves of all uncleanness; ask not, that ye may consume it on your lusts, but ask with a firmness unshaken, that ye will yield to no temptation, but that ye will serve the true and living God.

Birth is a miraculous thing. God is a God of miracles and He wants you to be a part of one.

These scriptures have parallels to visualizing. First, enlist the help of the Lord. Second, know what you want. Third, keep the picture in your mind. Fourth, do not doubt.

## Section 3

Visualizing can be a very effective tool, particularly when coupled with prayer. Your brain is more incredible than the finest computer. Heavenly Father created us after His own image. We have the capacity to grow and learn and become like Him.

Our subconscious mind remembers everything. It can trigger the same bodily response each time the same thing happens. Think of eating a lemon. Your mouth can begin puckering and/or watering just thinking about eating a lemon. What you think and what you believe is very real to your subconscious mind. This is why the saying is true that what you think about, you do.

Crimes are committed in the mind well before the actual act is done. On the other hand, people who experience success, whether spiritually, physically or mentally, believed and thought to be the person they became long before they accomplished the deed.

Your body readily complies with the commands of your mind. It is an amazing relationship. Imagine how quickly a baseball player's mind calculates to help him catch a ball. It has to know how far the ball will travel and if it will curve or fly a straight path. It has to tell the legs how fast to run to make it to the proper point on time. It has to tell the arms how far to stretch and the wrists how to bend and the fingers how to grasp.

If you have ever tried to teach a young child how to catch a ball, you know this ability comes from much repetition. First, you start perhaps with a balloon that falls more slowly and is easier to catch. Then you try a large, light ball. You show the child how to hold his hands out. Many are the times that his hands are too close to his face, or too far apart. Next you teach him how to catch a ball that doesn't land directly in his hands. You have to show him to watch the ball coming and move his hands to where the ball will come. Next, you have him catch a ball that he has to run for to catch. This sounds complicated, but most everyone learns to do it. It is pretty incredible to think about.

How did the child learn to do it? By repetition! Repeating it over and over until his mind knew exactly what to tell the body to do to catch any ball that came his way, whether fast or slow, spinning or straight, lobbed in the air, or coming right at him.

This is the exact concept you can use in teaching your subconscious mind how to tell your body to prepare for the coming of your baby. You can adapt your picture to the way you would like it to be. In chapter six, I have included a basic scenario of what could be expected throughout labor and delivery. You can use this as a guide to help you develop your own visual picture. You will want to include as many details as you can in your visualization to make it very real to your mind.

Some things that you can put into your visual picture include, but are not limited to the following: See yourself walking around in early labor, keeping in control. As the contractions become stronger, you see your supportive coach there to help you. You see yourself completely relaxed between contractions. When another one comes, your mind instructs your body to work with the contraction. Picture the muscles doing their job, working to bring your baby to you. You remain relaxed in all places except the contracting uterine muscles. No facial tension, relaxed arms and legs, etc. You are in control. You allow the uterus to contract and you remain relaxed so that the uterus can do its job uninhibited. You imagine the cervix effacing properly and dilating as it should. You picture the baby's head moving down the birth canal. Your body is stretching, stretching, widening to accommodate the baby's head. As the baby's head crowns and you feel the great pressure, your perineal area expands more and allows the baby through. As soon as the head is out, the rest of the baby follows quickly out as you keep ready and work with the contractions. You see yourself having Divine help when you need it.

If you will practice visualizing, this will be remembered by your subconscious mind. When the happy day arrives, your mind will be prepared to tell the body what it needs to do. This principle works. Your mind will recognize what is happening as soon as labor starts and you can remember to act the way you told yourself to act.

Visualize the birth as often as possible. At night before going to sleep is a very good time to do this, because then you will think about it as you are falling asleep.

If you think badly of your labor, and doubt that you can do it, you are right. On the other hand, if you think in positive terms, knowing that Heavenly Father and His angels will help you and your baby, that is also true. No matter what situation comes up, He can guide you. If you are prepared, you will have a good spiritual experience because you have trusted in Him. He can guide you to anything you might need to know prior to, or during your labor.

Let's say you are running a mile or more and feel like you can't go on, you give yourself a pep talk and ask God to help give you strength to finish the race. You can do it, and you do! The same is true of the birth experience. You can visualize. You can relax. You can eat well. You can be positive. You can stay in control. You can. You can. You can. He is there to help you. You are His daughter.

## Section 4

Maintaining a positive, happy attitude helps you to feel physically better and steers your thoughts in the right direction.

It is impossible to continually dwell on worries and be free of fear. Fear is not conducive to a positive, spiritual birth experience.

Being "stressed out" saps your body of needed B vitamins. A mind able to be calm and relaxed enhances the body's use of B vitamins.

Sometimes I think it is easier to remember not to allow ourselves to "stress out" when we have an extra reason to do so. If I know I will receive an immediate negative consequence for doing something, I am not likely to do it. For instance, I am not going to go and eat an item that I am allergic to, no matter how good it looks because I don't want the reaction that would come from eating it. If I know that dwelling on my worries could be harmful to my baby, I am more likely to watch my thoughts for his sake than I would be for my own sake.

Whatever you allow into your mind stays with you and makes you the person that you are. I have heard of the mind being compared to a stage with an ongoing play that you are in charge of. If someone or something undesirable is placed on the stage, you have the prerogative to allow it to remain, or to get rid of it. If there are evil people (negative thoughts) coming on to your stage, you must invite your fully armed righteous people (positive thoughts) to come to the stage in greater and greater numbers until the evil has departed.

Singing hymns, reading an uplifting book or praying are also good ideas for removing negative thoughts.

Section 5

Relaxation. Do you have difficulties relaxing? Do you need to de-stress? Do you need a little time for just you?

It is well worth the effort to <u>practice</u> relaxing. If you can take just a few minutes a day to practice, that is good. Practicing once at night before bedtime and once during the day is better. While you practice relaxing, it is also a good time to work on your visualization. As soon as you get yourself completely relaxed, you can go over your birth plan in your mind.

Relax? That is a joke, you say? I have other kids, you say? The good news is that they can actually help with the training! Yes, it is nice to be able to catch your relaxation time while they nap or are otherwise conveniently occupied, but if you can relax amidst commotion, you can learn to be a real pro! I am serious when I say this, because, chances are fairly good that something will come up when you are in real labor that makes it difficult for you to maintain control. So, if you have practiced relaxing in less than pristine conditions, you have an advantage.

I have found a few things that help me completely relax. If you can find what works well for you, you will fare much better during labor. If you are able to completely relax, it gives your hardworking body a break.

As hard as it is for me to remember this, I can conquer more tasks when I take a relaxation break than if I try to just work, work, work and take no breaks. This is true with everyday tasks, as well as with childbirth. You have to allow your body to rest between contractions!

Here is one relaxation technique.

First, I find a favorite classical music album to listen to. Sometimes playing the same music during labor is nice because music will often remind you of what you were doing at the time you last heard it. Thus you can remember how serene you felt as you relaxed.

I lay down on my bed after starting the music. Sometimes I could talk my husband into massaging my arms and legs. This can help relax tense muscles. Next, I would wiggle my toes and feet. Then I would relax them. To check if they were relaxed, it should seem almost as if they (my toes) weren't there, as in –did not exist. No twitching, no urge to scratch an itch, no desire to move any muscle in them. After that, I wiggle my legs and bend the knees a bit. Then relax them completely, trying again to come to the point where they were hardly noticeable.

I would do this with each part of my body, all the way up to my head. The face can sometimes be tricky. No tension whatsoever should show on the face.

Sometimes having someone check on you after five minutes is a good idea. Having someone picking up your arm and then dropping it, can be an indicator of the amount of tension left in your arm. Sometimes, someone can just look at you and tell if you have any visible stress.

Invariably the times when I wasn't completely relaxed was when I hadn't relaxed my mind. If the mind isn't relaxed, it just doesn't count as much!

In order to completely relax, I needed to empty my mind of my worries and think about something awesome, lovely, wonderful or soothing. I needed to let the beautiful music completely envelope me. I call it "shutting down my brain", kind of like getting a computer ready to shut off.

One of the best relaxing positions is to be on your back with a pillow under each leg and one under your head as well. Sometimes one under the knees is nice too. As pregnancy progresses, it is more comfortable to be only partially reclined rather than flat on your back.

Sometime during the day, try to shut down your mind for a few minutes. Put your feet up too. Even if just for five minutes. Your body will appreciate it. Take a few nice, big deep breaths too.

Another reason for practicing relaxation is that relaxing keeps the adrenalin flow down. The more anxious or apprehensive we feel the more adrenalin in the blood stream. This causes the red blood vessels to tighten. When they tighten, it restricts the amount of oxygen that gets through. The heart will also beat faster and your muscles will tighten. If your muscles tighten, your labor will slow down. It is harder for that baby to come out if you are resisting the birth.

If you know how to relax yourself, you relieve a lot of pressure from your mind during the labor and delivery. Also, relaxed muscles will dilate more easily. Your experience will be more rewarding if you learn to quickly relax yourself. You can rest between contractions. You can give your body a break.

## Section 6

Let me share a few thoughts on breastfeeding the baby.

Breastfeeding has been proven to be the best nourishment for babies. Of course, who needs a scientist to tell them that God knew what He was doing all along. The first milk that the baby intakes is called colostrum. Colostrum is very important for baby's immune system.

On about the third day after birth, the regular breast milk starts to come in. As your body adjusts to the needs of your baby, your breasts may become extremely full and uncomfortable. There are a few things that can be helpful.

Probably the best thing to remember is that within 24 to 48 hours it will start getting better! The problem will resolve, even if it may feel at the time like it will go on forever.

Standing in the shower and applying light pressure with a comb or your hands can alleviate some of the pressure. Many women will find that just standing in the shower will cause milk to drain. If this is the case for you, allow the milk to drain freely. This will definitely take the pressure off.

If you are very engorged, (swollen and hot to the touch), here is another suggestion. This may sound bizarre, but if you are at this point, you feel willing to try anything! Take some fresh cabbage leaves and apply them to your breast, avoiding the nipple. The coolness of the cabbage feels wonderful and somehow the cabbage alleviates some of the pressure as well. I don't know why or how this works, but it does work. You can put a cold wet washcloth on your breast, but it doesn't have quite the same effect. Change the leaves out when they become wilted.

It has been said by many that you should wake the baby every two hours and get him/her to nurse to help you out. I have often scoffed at this because waking a newborn baby isn't as easy as it sounds! I didn't have a lot of luck with this method with most of my babies. I had a midwife explain some strategies to me that weren't foolproof, but very often did the trick. If you can get the baby to wake up and eat, that is your best method for relief. Lay the baby down in front of you. Stroke the bottoms of his bare feet. Then undo his clothing and rub the baby's bare back up and down. (This is what they do to entice a cry from the newborn right after birth.) Don't put the baby up to your breast until you have gotten a good little cry or two from him that signifies he is ready. If you do, chances are good that the baby will just fall back asleep the second he is cuddled into your arms. Give yourself permission to wake the baby every two hours for a day or two for your own sake and for the sake of the baby. The baby can sense when mother is upset and often follows suit! You can allow the baby to go for a little longer during the night if you want to.

During pregnancy, you can prepare for nursing by using Lansinoh, olive oil, and/or vitamin e oil. A month or two before your due date, rub one of those products on your nipples after you get out of the shower. This helps to toughen them up to help prevent soreness, cracking and bleeding when you first begin to nurse. Not everyone experiences this problem. It is a lot more likely to occur if you have flat or inverted nipples.

When you begin nursing your baby, it may hurt at first. You can apply Lansinoh lanolin cream to help soothe and heal your nipples. This is good to have on hand before the baby is born. Once you have started to form blisters, cracks or bleeding, it is harder to heal.

If your baby has trouble latching on, keep trying. Eventually the baby will get it. You can try holding the baby in different positions. Getting a couple of drops of milk into his open mouth can also help encourage the baby to keep trying. Try to point the nipple towards the roof of the baby's mouth in order for him to have the best opportunity to grasp it.

Even if you are having troubles with nursing your baby, remain calm. Being relaxed, although this may seem difficult, really is helpful. If you find yourself becoming uptight and/or frustrated, give yourself a talking to. Remind yourself to calm down and that you and the baby will make it work as you persist.

There are lactation consultants that may be able to help if you feel you need some extra help. The la leche league has been around for a long time as well. You can find a lot of breastfeeding information from their website as well.

I have just tried to touch lightly on some problems that you may run into with breastfeeding. I do this not to discourage you, but to encourage you if you do happen to run in to any of these problems because breast milk really is the best thing for the baby. If you keep at it through the first week, things should be smooth sailing after that.

## Section 7

This section just contains a few more ideas from the miscellaneous category.

During early labor, drink lots of fluids. Yes, of course this will make trips to the restroom necessary, but it also gives you strength and prevents dehydration. Also, if you refrain from using the restroom and you have a long labor, you may experience problems afterward.

Keeping your stomach muscles pulled in can be a helpful thing during pregnancy. If you learn to hold your tummy in before pregnancy, you feel more able to "hold the baby up" in the last months of pregnancy. Many women feel as though they would like someone or something to help carry their swollen belly from about 6 months on. And, on the side of vanity, after the baby is born, it is nice to be able to suck your tummy in to give yourself a more slender appearance.

Try Kegel exercises throughout your pregnancy. These are good for keeping bladder control and strengthening those muscles. To do this, one simply pretends to need to use the bathroom but isn't able to do so. At least, this is the description of how you know which muscles to tighten and relax. These can be done several times throughout the day.

## Chapter VI:   Step by Step Guide: Summing It All Up

    I.       Pre-pregnancy
         a.  Build up a healthy body
         b.  Prayerfully invite children to your family
         c.  Find a good doctor or midwife

    II.      During Pregnancy
         a.  Continue to use healthy habits
         b.  Visualize the birth of your baby
         c.  Practice Relaxation
         d.  Let doctor or midwife know what you are wanting to have happen at your birth

    III.     Labor & Delivery
         a.  Pray for any needed inspiration to be given to yourself and those in attendance at the birth
         b.  Stick to your game plan --Remember what you visualized
         c.  Allow complete relaxation of your body, including your facial features
         d.  Focus on the miracle

While every birth will be slightly different, here is a basic scenario of what you might expect to happen.

*Early in the morning at 3:00 a.m. you wake up.  Being a little groggy, you think you probably might as well use the* bathroom since you are up. After your bathroom trip, you snuggle back up under your covers and go back to sleep. At 3:30 a.m. you find yourself awake again. Drat! Soon you are asleep again, only to be awakened once again at about 4:00 a.m. Your mind is a little more alert now and you realize that perhaps this might mean something. Sure enough, at 4:30 a.m. you notice your stomach begin to become very hard and your muscles are tightening. No wonder you keep waking up! At 4:45 you see that it is happening again. Could this be it?? When it happens again at 5:00 a.m., you decide it might be a good time to wake up your husband to share the news.

As soon as he is awake enough to figure out what you are talking about, the two of you begin to time contractions. You walk around a bit, talk, maybe grab a piece of toast and juice. Soon, you can see that the contractions are fairly rhythmic, coming every ten minutes. You decide to call the midwife. She lets you know she will be over soon. (If you are going to the hospital, you call the doctor when you are about 6 to 7 minutes apart and depart for the hospital when he gives you the go ahead shortly thereafter.)

The midwife arrives and checks the position of the baby and also lets you know that you are dilated to a 3. The midwife will stay at your home until the baby comes. She will be with you each step of the way. (If you go to the hospital, nurses will check on you intermittently and call the doctor when the impending birth is very near.)

*As the contractions get closer together, you find that you want to sit down in a semi-reclined position. Now is the time that you need to have a more concerted focus on what your body is doing. You get yourself as comfortable as possible, your husband helps prop pillows up where you want them. You go into a state of relaxation. Just as you practiced, you check each part of your body for signs of tension. First, you make sure your toes are relaxed, all the way up to your eyes.*

*As a contraction comes, you shift your focus from thinking about being relaxed to thinking about what your uterine muscles are doing. In your mind, you can see the muscles contracting and moving the baby towards the birth canal. As the contraction eases, your thoughts move away from thinking about muscles tightening and releasing. Instead, you focus on completely emptying your mind, so that only relaxation is taking place in between contractions.*

*With each contraction, your mind is allowed to pay attention to what the contracting muscles are doing, and also your mind wills the rest of your body to remain in a state of relaxation. This makes it so that all the work being done by your body is focused on the concentrated effort of the contraction. It makes it much more effective. No part of your body is tensing against the birth of the baby. Everything is allowed to happen naturally.*

*Of course the contractions become stronger and stronger. Each one taking you one step closer to holding your baby in your arms, but each stronger contraction also requires more mind work for you to keep yourself relaxed. Your husband encourages you by letting you know how well you are doing. If he notices you struggling, he helps you get back on track in whatever way is best for you. Perhaps he reminds you of your ability to relax each body part. Perhaps he lets you know that your body is doing what it is supposed to and that you are doing a good job keeping in control.*

*If you feel yourself needing help to remain in control, don't hesitate to ask for it. Your husband, your midwife or others in attendance may be able to be inspired with just what you need to hear in order to continue to remain in control. God will provide you the help you need in some way.*

*Soon you can feel the baby entering the birth canal and you sense the need to "bear down". This means that your body is telling you to gently push the baby down the birth canal. You do so very gently and under the guidance of the midwife or doctor. You picture your pushing efforts helping the baby to glide down the canal pathway.*

*When you are informed that the baby's head can be seen, this is a great encouragement to you. As the baby's head is crowning, you stop pushing. You may feel a burning sensation as your body expands to allow the head through. In your mind you picture your perineal area expanding as widely as it needs to for allowing the baby's head to be born. Your midwife may help in this with a little olive oil massage to make the transition easier. She may perhaps gently move your skin over the head if need be.*

*Next, the baby's shoulders are ready to come. You have been able to catch a glimpse of the baby's head, so you know how close you are to holding the baby. So, you work with your body to help the shoulders come out. Once the shoulders are out, the rest of the baby just slides out quite fluidly.*

*You feel elated that your baby is here! In a few more contractions, the placenta is out and you are free to enjoy your new baby completely.*

*A feeling of euphoria sets in as you cradle your newborn baby in your arms for the first time. You are sure there is nothing this side of heaven that could possibly compare with this moment. Even though your body is tired, your mind is completely invigorated as you bask in the warmth and love of your many blessings.*

Chapter VII: Healthy Snack Ideas

1. Make up your own trail mix

2. Thinly slice apples and sprinkle with pumpkin pie spice

3. Make Anthills ... by pressing in a few raisins in the top of a healthy muffin.

4. Dip various fruits in vanilla yogurt.

5. Make Ants on a Log by spreading peanut butter in a celery stalk and topping with raisins or currants.

6. Lightly sprinkle flour tortillas with water, sprinkle over cinnamon and sugar and bake at 400 until slightly crispy.

7. Use bamboo skewers to make Fruit Kabobs or Vegetable Kabobs. Try a fruit or veggie you have never tried before.

8. Make homemade popsicles. You can make any flavor imaginable that way...
-Grind up pineapple and bananas in the blender

-Use any flavor juice

-Add blueberries to juice before freezing

-Try any of the fruit drinks from this book

9. Melt Pepper-Jack cheese in flour tortillas in the microwave.

10. Vegetables and dip. (Always a winner!) Try different flavors of dip. Dill weed, garlic salt and lemon juice mixed in sour cream or nonfat plain yogurt is great. Chili powder, cumin, garlic salt and onion powder make a great Mexican dip.

11. Add garlic and onion to cream cheese. Serve with crackers, pretzels and veggies.

12. Have fruit starting to spoil? Cut off blemishes, puree in blender, layer in a dish with ice cream or yogurt.

13. Frozen Mango chunks are a favorite treat.

14. Chips and salsa

15. Rice and Ice Cream!  Reheat leftover rice if you have some, top with ice cream and cinnamon. Tastes like rice pudding, only surprisingly yummier!

16. Stuff Mini Taco Shells with cheese and various veggies and olives.  Serve with salsa for dipping.

17. Cut up melons for a fruit salad.

18. Cut up any other fruits, and or berries for an entirely different fruit salad.

19. Try bagels or toast with a variety of jams, honey, and spreads to try out.

20. Build your own open face sandwich. Be creative. Try some of these:

| | |
|---|---|
| Cucumbers | Radishes |
| Pickles | Mayo |
| Mustard | Dill |
| Chives | Peppers |
| Tomatoes | Cold boiled potatoes |
| Lettuce | Salad dressing |
| Cream cheese | Grated carrot |
| Raisins | Red onion |

## *Mom's Great Grated Apple Salad*

(My kids named this one.)

5 med. Apples-grated

1 can fruit cocktail (NO Sugar added)

Cinnamon to taste

Drain 2-3 TBS of juice from fruit cocktail and Drink or discard that juice.   Mix grated apples and fruit cocktail together in a medium size glass bowl.  Sprinkle with cinnamon and stir.  Refrigerate or serve right away.

## *Crackerjacks*

8 quarts popped corn

1 ½ cups honey

½ tsp. salt

1 ½ tsp. vanilla

¼ cup butter

1 cup raw or roasted peanuts

In a large saucepan, heat honey and salt over medium heat until hard crack stage.  Hard crack stage is when a few drops of the honey mixture dripped into a cup of cold water will make a strand of brittle candy that cracks when you try to bend it.  Take off heat and add butter, vanilla, and peanuts.  Stir well and pour over popcorn, mixing thoroughly to coat.  Spread on 2 cookie sheets to cool. Break into clusters

### Monkey's Delight

Popsicle or craft sticks

Bananas

Yogurt, any flavor

Shredded coconut, sweetened or unsweetened

Slice banana in half.  Insert Popsicle stick.  Dip in yogurt. Roll in coconut.  Serve.

### Whole Wheat Candy

1 cup butter

1 cup honey

1 ½ cups w.w. flour

1 cup peanut butter

nuts, coconut, sesame seeds

Melt butter, honey, and peanut butter.  Add flour.  Cook and stir a few minutes.  Add nuts, seeds, and coconut if desired.  Roll into balls.

### Any-flavor-no-ice-cream-but-delicious-shakes!

1 can evaporated milk

¼ cup fructose or honey, give or take a bit depending on desired sweetness and tartness of fruit.

More than 1 tray of ice cubes (enough to make it as thick as you like)

Approximately 1 tsp. vanilla

1 or more of the following:

3-4 peaches, 1 cup blueberries, 1 ½ cup strawberries, 2 bananas, ¼ cup carob, 4 TBS carnation malted milk powder, any other fruit you want or leave it vanilla flavored.

Put milk and fructose in blender. Slowly add rest of ingredients, preferably while blender is running (if you have a hole in top) Grind until smooth consistency. These really taste every bit as good as an ice cream shake.

### *Jungle Jumble*

1 20 oz can pineapple chunks, drained

1 cup grapes

2 bananas, peeled and sliced

1 red apple, chopped

1 orange, cut up

1 tsp. lemon juice

Put pineapple and grapes into a large bowl with lid. Add rest of ingredients. Put the lid on and "jumble" the fruit back and forth, upside down, until well mixed. Serves 4

### *Monkey Muffins*

1 cup wheat flour

2 ½ tsp. Baking powder

¾ cup oats

¼ tsp. salt

¼ tsp. baking soda

3 Tbl. Honey

½ cup milk

1 egg white

1 Tbl. Oil

2 mashed ripe bananas

Preheat oven to 400. Combine dry ingredients. Add egg white, but don't mix. Add honey, milk, oil, and bananas to the flour mixture. Stir with a fork until just moistened. Fill Muffin cups 2/3 full. Bake about 18 to 20 minutes (till slightly browned). Makes 12 muffins

### *Tutti-frutti Treat*

½ med. Red apple, peeled, chopped

1 cup applesauce, unsweetened

¼ cup crushed pineapple, drained

1/8 cup raisins

¼ tsp. cinnamon

6 Tbs. Vanilla yogurt

Put apple in medium sized bowl. Add all but yogurt. Chill or eat it now. Serve topped with 1 tablespoon yogurt. 6 servings.

### *1 Potato, 2 Potato 3 Potato, 4*

2 medium <u>baked</u> potatoes

2 Tbs. Apple juice

1 tsp. Seasoned salt


Slice potatoes lengthwise into 4 wedges.  Place in a large bow.  Add apple juice.  Stir until all potatoes covered with juice evenly.  Transfer wedges to another bowl, add seasoning, and stir till each wedge is covered.  Lightly grease a cookie sheet.  Don't let the wedges touch each other.  Bake for 7 minutes at 400 degrees.  Turn the wedges over and cook for 7 more minutes.  Eat.

### *Indian Summer Salad*

½ cup crushed pineapple, drained

2 cups shredded carrots

¼ cup raisins


Mix altogether.  Can serve on plate over a lettuce leaf.  Eat now or chill first.  Serves 2

### *Nuts Gone Crazy*

1 cup honey

½ cup peanut butter

1 tsp. vanilla

½ cup unsweetened shredded coconut

½ cup chopped almonds

1 cup oatmeal

Chopped walnuts to roll candies in

Cook honey over medium heat until it reaches the soft ball stage. To test for soft ball, drip a few drops of the cooked honey in a cup of very cold water. Gather the honey into a ball with your fingers. A soft ball will flatten without you pressing on it. Take off heat and add vanilla. Cool and add peanut butter, almonds, coconut and oatmeal. Scoop out tablespoonfuls and form into round balls. Roll in chopped nuts. Chill.

### *Tropical Slurpee*

1 6 oz can frozen orange juice concentrate

1 12 oz can crushed pineapple with juice

2 trays of ice cubes

In blender, process o.j. and pineapple until smooth. Add ice cubes a few at a time and blend well.

### *EZ Cinnamon Rolls*

1 loaf frozen bread dough

Oil spritzer

Cinnamon

Raisins

Honey

Chopped nuts

Allow dough to thaw.  Roll out to a rectangular shape.
Spray with oil.  Sprinkle with cinnamon, raisins, and nuts.
Squirt honey over it.  Roll it up from the long side.  Cut into
about 12 pieces.  Lay swirly side up in a greased pan.  Let
it rise until doubled.  Bake at 350 for about 15 to 20
minutes or till golden.  (Yes, it is sticky when you cut it and
put in pan.)

### *Molasses Cookies*

1 cup ww flour
1 cup white flour
1 tsp. baking soda
½ tsp. salt
½ tsp. ginger
1 tsp. cinnamon
1 stick butter
1/3 cup dark brown sugar
1 egg
½ cup molasses
¼ cup milk or water

Beat the butter till fluffy.  Add Sugar, egg and molasses.
Add 1 cup flour and sprinkle spices, salt, and soda over the
flour.
Then mix together at low speed.  Add the milk and the rest
of the flour.  Drop by the teaspoon onto greased cookie
sheets, about 2 inches apart.  Bake for 8 to 10 minutes at

375 degrees. Cool on wire rake. Makes 48 small or 24 larger cookies.

## *My Favorite Blueberry Muffins*

1 cup whole wheat flour

½ cup white flour

2 tsp. baking powder

¼ tsp. salt

1 egg

½ cup milk

½ cup honey

¼ cup oil (or ½ of it applesauce)

1 tsp. lemon zest from peel

¾ cup frozen blueberries

Mix dry ingredients except white flour. Add wet ingredients in hole in center of dry ingredients. Mix wet ingredients together before stirring altogether into the dry. In a small bowl, mix blueberries and white flour. Add to muffin batter. Don't stir too much. Should be lumpy. Fill paper bake cups 2/3 full and bake at 400 for 18 to 20 minutes or until lightly browned on top. Makes about 12

## *Strawberry Smoothies*

3 cups milk

2 large frozen bananas

1 cup frozen strawberries

1 tsp. vanilla

Put milk and vanilla in blender.  While running, add bananas and strawberries until the mixture is the consistency of a milkshake. Serves 4. Use frozen peaches, berries or other fruit for variation.

## Honey Fruit Bars

1 ½ cups peanut butter

1 cup honey

¾ cup brown sugar

5 cups raisin bran cereal

1 cup raisins and /or dates

Grease a 9 X 13 inch pan.  In a medium saucepan, combine peanut butter, honey, and sugar.  Bring to a boil over medium high heat.  Stir constantly.  Remove from heat and stir in remaining ingredients.  Turn the mixture into the prepared pan.  Using waxed paper, press the mixture down to distribute evenly in the pan.  Cool for 15 minutes.  Cut into 18 bars.

## *Fruit Smoothies*

1-2 cups frozen strawberries

1 cup frozen peaches

½ cup or less frozen blueberries

2-3 cups of apple, grape, or other juice

Other fruit, i.e. Oranges, lemon, banana

In a blender, grind up about ¼ of the ingredients at a time. When you have it all processed, it should be smooth and fairly thick. Use your imagination and vary the amounts of the types of fruits. For a thicker, dessert type drink, use more frozen fruits. For a breakfast type drink, use more fresh fruits. Do not use too many blueberries or bananas because their flavors will overpower other flavors. It really is difficult to have this turn out badly. It is hard to beat for super taste, healthy treat and family pleaser.

### *Cougar Crunch—A BYU favorite.*

| | |
|---|---|
| Peanut butter | Wheat germ |
| Honey | Oats |
| Wheat flour | Coconut |
| Other flours | Vanilla |
| Millet | Cornmeal |
| Any kinds of nuts | raw granola |
| Sunflower seeds | Sesame seeds |

Peanut butter, honey, and flour makes up the base of this. Add the rest and form into balls. You have done well if it is not too sticky and tastes good to you. Adding raisins and other dried fruit makes it Gorilla Grub. This is a great tasting way to eat raw nuts.

## *EZ bean dip for chips*

2 cans chickpeas (garbanzos)

About 1 cup salsa (Pace Picante is good)

2-3 TBS chopped fresh cilantro (opt.)

Grind till smooth in blender a bit at a time. Serve with chips, crackers and/or celery sticks.

## *Tips & Tricks*

➢ You can use ½ wheat and ½ white flour and most all cookies, etc. will turn out tasting just as tasty and work just as well as if you use all white. Also this makes it better for you.

➢ Freeze bananas in a Ziploc bag to have on hand for shakes, etc. Be sure to peel them first.

Chapter VIII: Baby #1

I am writing these pregnancy and birth stories in the hopes that it can help show what I learned through each one. Hopefully, those who read these words whether they are giving birth to baby #1 or baby #10 this time, will find some true helps from my experiences. Perhaps you can see yourself in some of my words.

Baby #1 was born a year, almost to the day, after our wedding. Looking back at journal entries, it is hard to believe how impatient I was to have a child. A year is nothing. I can see that now in retrospect. At the time, I wrote that I sometimes wondered if perhaps no child wanted to come to me as a mom, so insecure was I. I had fears and doubts. I can laugh now, because I can see that I was fretting and worrying and wondering right through the beginning stages of pregnancy. Little did I know what God had in store for me over the years.

Five months into my marriage, I discovered that I was expecting. I was so thankful. But, still being in the newlywed blissful stage, I commented "I must certainly admit that marriage is better than pregnancy!"

I prayed, "I hope and pray that I am giving him or her the proper nourishment so the baby will be healthy and strong. I hope and pray too that I will always remember how thankful I am for this little miracle, even mostly when I feel sick, nauseous and hungry all day. And also when I get big and round and get backaches and can't get out of chairs and whatever troubles come. I am so excited at the prospect of having a little one to take care of and hold. One who will have many of my characteristics and many of Kevin's and also some of his/her own."

I tried to imagine "what an offspring of Kevin and I will look like. I imagine a very beautiful baby with blonde hair, big blue eyes, probably very alert and not wanting to miss out on anything." This turned out to be the complete truth!

I was so excited. My family was excited. This was the first grandbaby on my side of the family. Word spread quickly.

I became astonished at how much I could eat. "I get hungry so fast!" I was so amazed at what I could pack away that I wrote a list of what I had eaten that day and was still in need of a bedtime snack.

"A few graham crackers

1 banana

A small bowl of familia hot cereal

A few slices of pickles

1 ½ cans of tuna fish

A few peach slices

A bowl of strawberries

A bowl of boysenberries

A good sized piece of homemade bread

Lots of almonds

Au Gratin potatoes

A few cucumbers

A natural foods candy bar

¾ cup of yogurt"

I decided to give up chocolate for two reasons. First is that it probably wasn't the best of things to nourish a baby with. Second, I like chocolate entirely too much, so I decided removing the temptation completely was probably a good idea anyway.

I put on 8 lbs in two months. I also chronicled my morning sickness episodes, of which there were 8. I thought I had gotten off fairly easily since my Mother had vomited 6 to 8 times a day sometimes.

I was grateful to be able to get my house cleaned up and keep it somewhat that way. (I should have enjoyed that while it lasted!)

I wrote a description of hunger during pregnancy, claiming that it was like as if you were fasting but the intensity is quadrupled.

What a joy it was to feel the baby kicking! "It is so fun to know that something is for sure alive in there."

I started reading pregnancy books and felt I needed to do more. I learned about Raspberry leaf tea and nettle tea. I determined to do better with taking my calcium and iron.

Closer to my due date, I started counting down the days. "In just 29 days, our baby is supposed to be here. It is still hard to comprehend even though our house is getting more baby things in it and my stomach is poking out and someone in there keeps moving around and kicking. We can't even imagine what it will be like to have a baby in our home, but we know it will be wonderful and also a lot of work. We are praying and trying to learn to be good parents, but we really don't know what we need to learn."

"We are trying to do those things that are best for our baby now, in the hospital, and afterwards. I am trying to eat well and take the things I should to give the baby the best chance possible to be good and healthy."

Finally, the big day arrived. Here's the story...

"I went to bed on Wednesday and did not sleep well from the very beginning. Trips to the bathroom and weird feelings in my lower tummy area kept me awake. I wondered what was going on. From 4:00 a.m. on, I started getting suspicious when I would get the pains about every 10 minutes or so. But, I kept thinking it couldn't be labor because I didn't think that was what it was supposed to feel like. At about 5:30, I asked Kevin if he was awake.

He said something that I interpreted to mean "sort of". He asked what was wrong.

I said, "I think we are going to have the baby today."

He said, "Are you serious?! I'm awake now!"

I called Mom at about 6:30 a.m. Still a bit sleepy, she jokingly asked, "What's the matter, are we having babies?" When I said I thought so, Mom had trouble believing it. In fact, she kept thinking I was probably just in false labor. She came to my house later and by 1:00 was pretty convinced.

At 2:00 we left for the hospital with contractions about 3 minutes apart. I was just hoping that I was progressing well enough that they wouldn't send me back home. I was dilated to 4 centimeters.

While Kevin went down to check me in to the hospital, our doctor came in to break my bag of waters. I said I didn't want him to. I don't think many people go against his "regular routine procedures" because he did not seem too happy with me. He said, "Well, whatever you want, but you are going to have a lot longer labor."

That was okay with me. I didn't want my baby to have any unnecessary stresses. He was going through a lot as it was.

We were very fortunate to have a really nice nurse. She gave some good advice. She told me, "You are in control" and also "concentrate on the breathing, not the contractions."

That was just what I needed to hear because I was feeling a bit out of control. I didn't know how to handle things. When she said that, I realized that she was right. I am in control. That helped so much.

From then on, my good coach, Kevin, talked me through every contraction and it gave me strength to endure and go on when I heard him tell me again, "you are in control."

Breathe in and out slowly and when I didn't, he gently chastened me. He was also generous with compliments when I did well.

My mother was there too, offering me a drink now and then. She had also placed her hand gently on my knee at some point. I mention this because I made her leave it there for some strange reason. I think it was because when she would move it, then I would notice something had changed and I would forget to focus on being in control. Instead I would notice the hand not being there anymore.

At around 5:30, Kevin and I were alone in the room. We heard a big "pop" sound and then I felt and heard water running. Kevin, being startled, stated the obvious, "I think your water broke, honey."

For some reason, that made me really happy. The nurse came and checked me shortly thereafter and found I was dilated to 10 cm. She then set up the room with things needed for the delivery and left again.

The doctor and the nurse came back at about 6:30. The doctor was not pleased that I didn't want an episiotomy.

When the baby was crowning, I was supposed to have stopped pushing so as to limit tearing. Neither Kevin nor I remembered this from the classes we had taken. Mom didn't remember either. The doctor didn't say a word. Because of this, I tore pretty badly and needed quite a few stitches. (In consecutive births, I never needed any stitches.)

Kevin kept coaching me and told me it would be just a few more pushes and the baby would be here. The doctor said that Kevin was wrong and it would probably be still quite some time. I chose to believe Kevin and happily the baby came within 10 minutes. What a relief it was to see that little baby come out. I could hardly believe I just had a baby.

Within a few minutes of the birth, the placenta was also out. The doctor told me I must take pitocin shot or I would bleed to death. I didn't take it.

After they cleaned him off a bit and wrapped him in a blanket, they gave him to me to hold. What a precious bundle! He was so cute! He was very, very healthy and strong. After everyone had held him, they took him to the nursery. I was left alone.

It would be 4 hours before I got my baby back. How long that would be, I thought. And it was.

While I was alone for a while, however, I was able to think about what had happened. First, I was extremely thankful to my Heavenly Father for sending such a beautiful, healthy, lovely baby boy.

I also thought how blessed I am to have such a good, loving, kind and compassionate husband. Kevin helped me more than he realized. He sat for many hours on that hard little stool without pausing for eating and only once or twice to stretch his aching back.

During my time alone, I also thought about how blessed I was to have strength and help sent from Heaven. Even though I saw no angels, I know they were present as they helped my little one and I make the transition from their presence to mine.

I thought how wonderful it was that God entrusted this special little soul to our care. I lay there with tears running down my face for a good half an hour thinking of my many wonderful blessings. Me, a child of God who would now have the opportunity to love and care for another tiny, precious child of God.

Chapter IX: Baby #2

My firstborn was just over five months old when I figured out for certain that I was expecting again. I knew I wanted to have a lot of children, so this wasn't something to be sad about. So, why did I spend a few weeks feeling depressed? I felt badly for my firstborn, for one thing. I couldn't continue to nurse him because my body was exhausted and milk production had slowed tremendously. He was still getting up several times at night. I worried that I wouldn't be able to give him what he needed. I wanted him to have mother's milk, which is the best thing for baby. I also didn't feel like I was ready to have another baby so soon. It didn't take long after prayer and conversation with Kevin to feel a relief and have a better outlook. I knew we were being blessed to have another baby. I knew we would love each precious little one that came to us. We just hoped the baby wouldn't arrive until after Kevin's finals!

We had no maternity insurance. This was not a huge problem, because we had already decided months ago, after much reading and studying, that we wanted to have our next child born at home. But, still, it was a bit of a concern in case it was needed.

So, we found an experienced midwife to assist in the birth. It was interesting to me to note that I didn't have to wait for a long period of time in a waiting room to see her.  And, when I did see her, it was for more than three minutes.  I learned that she wasn't interested in a lot of interventions, but would allow the birth to proceed naturally.

At 9:00 in the morning, we went to church.  Church lasted until noon.  I had a few contractions during church.  Once home, the contractions started coming closer together.  The midwife was called and she and her assistant came to spend the day with us.

I felt a little better prepared going in to this labor than I had with my first child.  I was glad I knew that I had some control over things.  During labor, my strategy was to block out actions going on around me and to fully concentrate on "not concentrating on the contractions".  That sounds pretty funny, but that is what I was doing.  I watched a clock with a minute hand.  This seemed very helpful to me because contractions rarely lasted over a minute, so I knew that when it got past the 30 second mark, the contraction would begin to subside.  I relaxed more for the last half the contraction.   My goal was to focus on the clock and not on the contraction.

I listened to Kevin coaching me through the contractions.  Kevin tried getting me to think of things other than the contractions by painting a word picture of a beautiful log home in the mountains surrounded by trees, streams and open areas.

Doing these things was more effective than what I had started doing with my first child. With him, I had had trouble figuring out what, if anything, I should do. I thought, initially, that my body was going to do what it was going to do and I had no idea what to do with my thoughts. After the nurse told me that I was in control, my thoughts began to become more positive, less worried and panicked.

At one point during labor, I was able to get into the bath tub and had warm water poured over me with each contraction. This really seemed to ease the force of the contraction. I stayed there for a while.

The contractions became harder. The baby was closer to arrival. I was in pretty much a sitting position for the birth. The baby was ready to come, but I was fearful of pushing because I worried about tearing again if I pushed at the wrong time. But, the midwife provided the needed coaching and encouraged me to push at the appropriate time. Then, when the baby was crowning, she told me to stop. It took only three total contractions from that point until the baby had completely emerged from the birth canal.

Kevin got to help the baby out. He also got to cut and clamp the cord. He was very glad at this extra participation in the birth. He didn't get to do that with our first.

I was able to hold the baby immediately. She was able to nurse before the midwife took her to weigh her, measure her, and otherwise check her over.

The little darling popped her tiny thumb in her mouth within minutes of having been born. Her brother, who was 11 ½ months old, came to see her. It was a tender moment. He ran out of the room and came back with a book that he proceeded to "read" to her.

It was nice. We were together as a family. We were home. I was in my own bed. No hospital food. A peaceful atmosphere. Love.

Chapter X: Baby #3

Tears. Lots of them. I definitely wanted to have another baby. But, already, again? How was I supposed to handle that many babies at once? Hadn't I "earned" a break from being pregnant for a little while? This baby was to arrive approximately one year after baby #2, and approximately two years after baby #1. Yikes!

Needless to say, mentally I didn't want to go through labor and delivery again so soon. I believe that this is what led to the problems I encountered for this birth.

We weren't able to calculate an exact due date for this baby. We had a pretty good idea, but time kept ticking by and the baby hadn't come yet. We really didn't anticipate the baby coming as late as he did. The midwife suggested that I might want to take something to promote the labor process. I wasn't too sure if I wanted to or not. We decided to pray for the baby to just come that night. If nothing happened by the next afternoon, I would take something because we really felt like the baby needed to come now.

At about 3:00 in the morning, I started having some contractions. I told Kevin when he got up for work that he probably should stay home. Shortly after he called and told his boss he wouldn't be coming in, the contractions stopped.

I had gone into false labor about 3 weeks before, so it was rather annoying to have the contractions stop again. I knew that God would make everything turn out alright; I felt that in my heart. But it was a discouraging start.

In the late afternoon, I started having contractions again. We called the midwife and she and her attendants started off to our house. By the time they got there, the contractions were nearly at a standstill again.

The midwife had dealt with similar situations before. She knew to give me some blue cohosh tincture, which is an herb that helps promote labor. She gave a little of this to me about every 15 minutes. This did the job. The contractions kept coming.

Since we were heading in to night time, we all laid down to get some rest. The problem was that I was able to go to sleep! So, the midwife or one of her attendants got the job of coming to wake me and give me more tincture every so often. Finally, it was enough to get some serious contractions to happen and keep happening.

I was glad because I felt I was doing quite well at keeping in control. Things weren't progressing very well, though. I had been in labor off and on for a very long time now—over 24 hours. The midwife broke the bag of waters because she said the bag was really tough. I was relieved that she did this because I thought that it would be no more than a half an hour before the baby would be here. My reasoning was that it took no longer than that with the other two.

I was getting frustrated because nothing seemed to be happening. I could not feel the baby moving down the birth canal as I could with the previous two. It felt like everything was at a standstill, except for the contractions. I kept trying to keep my mind in control, but I could hear them in the background saying something about a cervical lip. I had no idea what exactly that meant, but I figured it must have something to do with why the baby wasn't coming. I started having trouble keeping my mind in control. It was then I just verbally called out to God to help me. All who were in attendance kept reassuring me at that point that God and His angels were indeed helping.

Whenever I needed help again, I said the same thing and got the reassurance that gave me the strength I needed to keep going. Knowing that God was with me was what helped me through that last hour.

The midwife had one of her attendants working my cervix. Then, finally, the baby started moving down. When he started to crown, I felt fear that he was going to be too big and I would tear.

After such a long labor, when he was all the way out, I was more relieved than you can even imagine. They lay him immediately on my thigh and tummy. I was able to cradle him in my arms. It was such a wondrous feeling.

Then everything was worth it. There's nothing more precious and glorious than holding that newborn baby right after birth.

I found out what had been happening after the baby was born. When nothing was happening, it was because the cervix had created a lip up over the baby's head and he couldn't get past it. That is why it felt like his head was so big that I would tear. I did have a slight tear, but needed no stitches. That is why the attendant needed to work the cervix. In the end, the midwife had to help pull the cervical lip down the rest of the way to allow the baby to come through.

Looking back, I believe that I had been resisting what was imminent. My mind had told me many times how I wasn't ready for another birth yet and how much I didn't want to go through it. My mind was working against what my body was naturally trying to do.

This was a good learning experience for me because it made me want to see what I could do in the future to make sure my mind was better prepared before birth arrived. I promised myself I would be ready mentally when the next one came.

Even though the birth of baby #3 was difficult, I had to be so grateful to God for all the help I had in getting the baby here. I believe in miracles. As with every birth, this was a miracle; but I felt that I got a few little bonus miracles to help me along the way when I wasn't strong enough on my own.

Chapter XI: Baby #4

Kevin and I started considering having another baby. Baby #3 was two years old. About a month after having these thoughts, my mother convinced me to take a pregnancy test. Sure enough, it was positive! (Mother knows best?) Even though I didn't think I was expecting, I think God really knows best what we need in our lives. I was very happy and excited. My three children were excited when we told them. By the time the baby was to come, they would be ages almost 3, 4, and 5. They were going to love to help out. It would be good for all of us to have a little babe around.

We had moved and I found a new midwife. I was very pleased with the extra care and time she took with me at each appointment. She often gave me good encouragement and guidance.

The pregnancy itself was fairly uneventful. I did start a theme that would recur through consecutive pregnancies. I was told to get more protein, drink protein shakes, etc.

Once again, we were unable to have a great degree of accuracy in figuring out a due date. On the date that we initially stated for the due date, we had a lot of family in town for a family event. I became rather discouraged because I had about 20 relatives asking me daily if anything was happening!  They all wanted to see the baby before going back to their homes.

I had had Braxton Hicks contractions with this baby. Not bad ones, really, but enough to notice.  Not having had any with the other kids, I had thought a few times that I was going in to labor.  But, then nothing would come of it. I was feeling kind of embarrassed, because one would think that by baby number 4, you would know for sure if you were in labor!

The relatives all said that of course the baby would come the day after everyone had gone.  No such luck.  I was feeling stressed!

Finally, the day arrived! It came three weeks beyond our initial guess at the due date!

At about 5:00 a.m. I was starting to get mad at those dumb Braxton Hicks contractions that wouldn't let me sleep.  By 6:00 a.m. it dawned on me that if these were waking me up, there was probably something more to it! So, I went and timed them for an hour and then decided to wake Kevin at 7:00 a.m.

After another half an hour, we decided it was time to call the midwife.  The contractions were about 10 minutes apart.  We called my Mom as well, so she could make it to the birth.  She had a 90 minute drive.

We called Kevin's sister who was to take the kids until the new one arrived. Kevin's sister's husband came and left with the kids at about 9:30.

No sooner had we called everyone that needed to get called, than my contractions jumped to every 3 to 4 minutes! Things were happening so very fast. I became a little panicked because things weren't following the pattern that I had come to expect from previous births. The contractions were so close together and hard so early in the labor process.

Kevin's Dad came over to assist Kevin in giving me a blessing. After the blessing, I determined to believe every word Kevin said. And, I really did. Kevin kept telling me to concentrate. Even in the middle of labor, I found his statement humorous because he didn't tell me what to concentrate on! So, I chose to concentrate on him. With each contraction, I looked at Kevin and expected him to encourage me through it as I tried to just breathe through the contraction. He talked me through each one.

My Mom finally showed up by about 9:30 or 9:40 a.m. She had been slowed down by construction. When she arrived, the midwife hurried her in, saying that I was just waiting for her. I believe this is probably true because I was a bit more at ease when she did arrive.

Within minutes of Mom's arrival, it was time to help push the baby down the birth canal. The water had not broken yet, but baby was coming. As soon as the baby crowned, it took only a few contractions for the baby to emerge. He was born "in the caul". This just meant that the water sac didn't break. The midwife broke the sac after the baby was born. She told us it was a very rare occurrence for this to happen. She said he must be a very special baby.

Baby was born at 9:59 a.m. I was the first to notice he was a boy. We were all surprised at how much he weighed (8 lbs 13 oz) and at how long he was (21 ½ inches). I was able to hold him right away.

The delivery of the placenta was much easier than with the other three. Really, there wasn't much to it in comparison with the others.

I had had no afterpains with my firstborn. Only a minimal amount with my second born. I had quite a few with my third child. So, I was expecting to have a lot with my fourth. However, I had hardly any. I had many more with the third than with the fourth.

As it turned out, baby number four was my best birth experience yet. It was nice having such a short labor, even though it was hard to adjust in the beginning to it being different. I had more energy afterward. We determined that perhaps part of the reason the labor was so short was that I had taken an herbal remedy that was a cervix softener in order to help prevent what had happened with baby number three. In addition to that, I had taken an herbal 6 week formula that had some of the same ingredients in it. (That probably wasn't my smartest move—not recommended!) But, then again, now that I know this child (he is 12 at the time of this writing) it could have simply been the fact that this child hates change, but when he does things, he does them very quickly! He probably was snug and cozy in my tummy and wanted to stay as long as possible, even though it drove me crazy to wait 3 weeks. Then, when he came, he did it in 1/3 of the time it had taken with the first two.

In my journal, I wrote that this child was such an "angel baby." He was a very good sleeper for a newborn. By two days old, I had coaxed several smiles out of him—if my heart hadn't already been completely in love with him, those smiles would have done it. Yes, he was a very special baby. Oh how wonderful it is to have a newborn to love and hold. Boy, am I blessed.

Chapter XII: Baby #5

What a busy time of life. Lots of changes, not the least of which was to be a big move and job change. We sure did hope that this baby decided not to have a late arrival! As it turned out, baby came two days before his due date, giving me three weeks recuperation time before our out of state move.

I had a lot of Braxton-Hicks contractions two days before his arrival. I thought it might be working into something more, but I went to bed at about 11:00 p.m. and fell promptly asleep and the contractions disappeared.

The next day, the same thing seemed to be happening. I had pretty strong contractions off and on all day that were stronger than the day before.

By 8:00 that night, when Kevin came home, we decided to time them. They were rather irregular, but came on average about 6 to 7 minutes apart. We decided to call the midwife. We had the same midwife as with the last baby, but we had moved and she was 90 miles away. She arrived at about 10:30.

I was very embarrassed when my contractions had nearly stopped by the time she got there. I was only slightly dilated. The midwife was very kind and encouraging. She stayed until midnight and then determined it was time to go home. She said we all should go to bed and if I fell right asleep, then that just meant that what I had been experiencing was just practicing. And that was okay. It happens.

Sure enough, I fell right asleep, but I woke up at 3:30 a.m. with contractions that I could feel in the inner center. This is a sign of the "real thing." I soon decided it was serious enough to wake Kevin.

We did some timing to make sure. After a few contractions, I knew I was really in labor this time. We called my poor midwife and she came back. (She didn't get much sleep that night, I am sure!)

I had spent much time visualizing this birth before it happened. I spent a lot of time practicing complete relaxation as well. These two things went hand in hand. I pictured myself concentrating on relaxation, meaning complete and total relaxation with no tension at all. I paid particular attention to my facial tension. I visualized having no tension going on in my body at all.

My visualization efforts paid off quite well. Whenever a contraction would come, I concentrated only on making sure I was completely relaxed. I envisioned my uterine muscles working as they were supposed to work.

I did so well with concentrating on my relaxation, it was most often not evident to those present in the room, when I was having a contraction.

Kevin actually slept through most of my labor. I was so focused on relaxing, that it wasn't until very close to the birth that I needed his assistance. I would give his hand a quick squeeze as a contraction started. Mom, the midwife, and her assistant mostly left us alone, except checking in on us occasionally. As it came time for the birth, of course they stayed.

I was so very pleased that the laboring went just as I had envisioned, as far as being in control and very relaxed. It really took away a great deal of pain to be completely relaxed. I really think practicing relaxing helped a lot.

This baby had a rather large head and also shoulder distortia. This may be part of the reason why I had a hard time remaining in control during the pushing stage. But, I also didn't spend much time envisioning the actual delivery part of birth. I wondered if I could perhaps do some more studying to come up with a better method of remaining in control during the final stage.

As with baby number 3, my contractions never got regular. Sometimes I was able to sneak in a short, little nap between contractions. But, they didn't stop. I had a cervical lip with this baby, just as with baby number 3. This midwife was able to take care of the problem much more quickly and easily than the other midwife had been able to. Perhaps it wasn't as severe. Perhaps it helped because I had been so relaxed. I don't know for sure. They say it is very common to have a cervical lip with consecutive babies if you have had it before.

Once again, I was able to experience the wonderful miracle of holding a brand new baby in my arms. Nothing in the world can compare to that feeling. All the other kids were so anxious to see their new brother. Watching their faces as they held him so carefully was another tender moment. The three year old made up a couple of interesting names for him. All of them had a sense of wonder shining in their eyes. God is so good.

Chapter XIII: Baby #6

Once again, it was going to be time to welcome a new baby into the family. Baby #5 would be almost 5 years old when this one would arrive. Having 4 boys and 1 girl, our daughter was really hoping and praying for a little sister. Of course, Kevin and I were too.

I had been having some hypoglycemic type problems and we were a bit concerned about this. I felt pretty lousy for the first four months of pregnancy, but after that, I felt pretty well.

This baby was going to be born in the hospital. We were in a bit of a financial pinch at the time, yet we had excellent maternity coverage with our insurance. We were blessed to find a doctor that was very willing to allow us to have the kind of birth we wanted to have. He never rushed me through appointments. He always made me feel as though he had time for whatever questions or concerns I had and didn't have a problem with me not wanting a lot of intervention during labor and delivery.

Kevin's parents were in town and this darling baby decided to cooperate and show up while they were here.

The day started at about 5:00 a.m. with contractions coming about every 15 minutes. I hadn't had many Braxton-Hicks with this baby, so I was pretty sure I was in labor. I had the mucus plug show early on. This was unusual for me. In fact, I don't really remember ever noticing it with any of the other kids.

We called the doctor's answering service and explained what was going on. The person on the other end of the line asked if it was my first baby. When I told her it was number 6, she sounded nearly frantic and told me I must get to the hospital right away! Personally, I thought it was too early to go in. But, we did as I was told and got ready to go around 9:30.

When we got checked in to the hospital, one of the nurses checked me and I was hardly dilated. The contractions, however, continued steadily and regularly. So, we took a walk around the hospital corridors for a while. The nurse checked again, and still didn't find much progress.

Soon, the hospital staff was ready to send me home. I told Kevin that if they did release us, we would just stay in the parking lot, because it felt to me that now would be about the time that I should be thinking of coming in. The staff had us call and talk to our doctor. He asked me to tell how I was feeling and what I thought should happen. I told him what I had said to Kevin. So, he convinced the staff to let us just stay.

From that point on, I started having more contractions and they were coming closer together. I used the same methods of relaxation and visualizing that I did with baby #5.  Again, whenever a contraction would come, I concentrated only on making sure I was completely relaxed, right down to the muscles in my face.  I also envisioned my uterine muscles working as they were supposed to work.  I pictured them contracting and then releasing as the baby worked his/her way to and through the birth canal.

This method worked marvelously well again.  Being in tune with my body and working with it, rather than against it, or thinking of other things, really makes a huge difference in birth.

The nurses apparently were still having difficulty believing that my labor was going anywhere.  There were often several in the room and they were talking rather loudly to one another.  Kevin did a good job of asking them a few times to quiet themselves down and letting them know I needed a peaceful atmosphere.

Even though we were at the hospital, I didn't want to have all the common interventions.  We declined having an I.V.  We sited the fact that I had given birth five times before without needing a needle in my arm.  I also didn't want any drugs or enemas or whatever else they wanted to thrust in my direction.

One nurse volunteered to break the bag of waters. We told her no as well.  I wanted to concentrate solely on the birth of the child. I wanted the Spirit of the Lord to be there with me. I didn't pay much attention to the distractions going on around me. I let Kevin deal with anything that came up.

The contractions became harder, closer together and more lengthy. The doctor wasn't there yet. I could feel the baby moving down the birth canal. But, I could tell something wasn't quite right. At that moment, I felt a prompting in my heart telling me that the bag of waters needed to be broken. I didn't doubt this feeling, even though it seemed rather unusual to now request an intervention that I had turned down. In between contractions, I told Kevin what needed to happen. The nurse came and broke the bag.

This was definitely what needed to happen. All of a sudden the baby was free to move down the canal. The doctor showed up then and discerned the need to slip the cord up over the baby's head.

The baby's head was pressing down on the cord and also on the bag of waters, so it seems that that was preventing the birth from progressing. During the final stages of pushing, I simply made "motorbike" sounds with my mouth. I don't know why, but it seemed helpful at the time. From the time the doctor showed up until baby's arrival, was under 15 minutes.

One of the nurses that had been with us from the beginning, left shortly before the baby was born. She told us the next day that if she had known it was going to be such a short time until delivery, she would have stayed. She was rather disappointed. But, Kevin kept telling the nurses that I was in hard labor and the birth would be soon. None of them believed him. No one could act the way I was acting and actually be in hard labor. But it is true. I was and did and could.

Focusing on the spiritual aspects of birth, completely relaxing during contractions, visualizing all work!

When the baby came out, we were thrilled to discover that she was a girl! She was a little blue at first, but quickly recovered and I was able to hold her. Oh, how happy we were to have another precious daughter. And how well loved she would be by us and her siblings. Once again, this little one was the most precious, sweetest, perfect baby ever to be held in my arms. (Funny how one can say that each and every time.)

Our eleven year old daughter was beside herself with joy to the point of nearly disbelieving what we said when we told her she had a sister.

The eight year old was thoroughly disgusted to hear he had another sister. That was up until the moment that they got to the hospital and he took her in his arms. From that point on, he was in love. He didn't want anyone else to hold her. That was one of the most precious things I have ever seen, watching the change that came over him. You see, God's love really does shine through the eyes of a newborn baby.

Chapter XIV: Baby #7

Here we go again! It finally occurred to me to take a pregnancy test after several days of not being able to understand why I was so ravenously hungry, mildly nauseous, tired and needing to use the rest room every five minutes. You would think that I would have figured it out sooner, having gone through this 6 times already! Yes, I discovered I was expecting #7.

Our youngest is five years old. She is very excited about the new baby. She will be 5 ½ by the time the baby gets here.

The first few months of this pregnancy were spent feeling rather tired. I took frequent naps. Also, I felt somewhat nauseated for the first few months, but it wasn't extreme. It was actually more of an overall "gross" feeling more than true nausea. I didn't really feel like vomiting, but I struggled to eat and just generally didn't feel great.

The second trimester went quite smoothly. I managed to do quite a few things in addition to keeping up with all six kids. I wrote songs, worked on this book, snuck in some time to go out to lunch with friends, etc.

With this baby being due around the holidays, (New Years) I was anxious to get everything done before Christmas, just in case! Usually, my mindset has been to get certain things accomplished before the baby's due date. But, with this child, the date that fixed in my mind was Christmas day. Because of this, after Christmas day came and went, I started to get antsy. I had no more deadlines; the kids were on school break, no pressing issues. So, I turned into a bit of an emotional rollercoaster with tears, happiness, anger, melancholy, you name it, it showed up. Finally, I decided that the best thing for me to do was to do some things that required brainpower since scrubbing the tub and cleaning just didn't take my mind off things!

On the baby's due date, January 4th, in the morning, I had a tinge of bloody mucous show. I took this as a good sign. Not much really happened until late afternoon. At that time I started getting a little stronger contractions, but not enough to make me feel like "this is it!" I remembered the possibility that I could still be days away from delivery, but I was hopeful I wouldn't have to wait that long. By bedtime, it was evident that no baby would come on January 4th.

During the night, I had contractions that would wake me up frequently. I went to the bathroom most every time I woke up and continued to get more bloody show. By morning I was sure that the baby would be born on this day.

We called the midwife in the morning and let her know what was going on. At the time, contractions were a steady half hour apart.  She said to let her know when they were closer together before she was going to come over.

As long as I stayed in bed and relaxed, the contractions kept coming.  If I got up and moved around, the contractions would slow down.  This is the opposite of how things generally work.  Looking back on it all, I am pretty certain that I know what was happening.  When I was up and around, I started focusing on things other than the birth.  I worried about what everyone else possibly wanted to have happen.  I was worrying about my other six kids that were to be farmed out to five different people's houses.  This was silly of me, but I couldn't seem to stop myself from it.

When I would lie back down in bed and relax, I would remind myself that the birth of this baby was between God, me and the baby.  Nothing was more important than that.  As I reminded myself of this, my body was able to relax and do its job.

In the early afternoon, we called the midwife back when the contractions were 10 to 12 minutes apart.  She said she would want to come when they were about 5 minutes apart.

The kids started to head off to various friends' houses.  The house got very still and quiet.  By about 3:00 in the afternoon, the contractions were about 6 to 7 minutes apart.  I got up, as suggested by the midwife, and moved around, trying to get things going more. As had happened before, the contractions slowed again.

By 6:00 they were back to 11 to 12 minutes apart. I decided I would walk around the house until 6:30. As I walked, I had maybe 3 contractions. None of them were very good ones. While I walked, I did some thinking. I reminded myself again that this was between God, me, and the baby. I told myself that I was just going to relax and not worry about if the baby was coming today or in a few days. By 6:30, I had convinced myself that as bedtime approached, I would just go to bed and sleep. If something decided to happen, it would, if not, then I wouldn't worry about it. If I was up 15 times in the night with contractions again, so be it. Maybe the baby would come the next day.

In this frame of mind, and with contractions nearly at a standstill, I sat down in a comfortable chair near Kevin who was watching a football game. He wanted to be helpful, but there really wasn't much for him to do except possibly time contractions. So, I just said, "'kay" when one would start and nod my head when it stopped. We continued on in this manner for a half hour or so until Kevin interrupted me to say that my contractions were coming every five minutes.

We had updated the midwife on what was going on at about 6:00. She said she would just come over at about 7:30 or 8:00 to check and see how things were going regardless of what was going on. She thought that might give me a bit of peace of mind whether the contractions were still slow or had sped up by then.

It was closing in on 8:00 and I told Kevin I needed to go use the bathroom, but I thought the midwife would be there any time, so I thought I would wait until she got there so I only needed to get up once in going down to the bedroom. He told me not to worry about that and just go. I didn't really need to be worried about getting up again if I didn't want to.

The midwife got there about 8:30 and I was propped up with pillows, sitting on the bed. She patiently checked the baby's heart tones with the fetal scope and monitor, felt the position of the baby's body and took my pulse and blood pressure. At about 9:00 she checked to see how dilated I was. I was at about a five.

Being at a five told me, intellectually, that I probably had at least a couple of hours before birth. So, I thought I should probably get up and use the restroom one more time while they changed the sheets in preparation for the birth.

On the way to the bathroom, I had to stop and work through a rather strong contraction. Kevin was with me then coaching me. It is hard to completely relax while in a standing position, so I felt the effects of that contraction full force. Kevin left the bathroom to go help change the bed.

The midwife was calling her assistant and then helped Kevin finish up. In the meantime, I had a couple more very intense contractions. I kept telling myself that I could relax, that I could do this. I had to be okay because I was by myself with no one helping me along at that time. I stood up to make my way back to the bedroom as Kevin came back in to check up on me.

I stopped in the doorway as another very strong contraction came on. I was thinking in my mind that if I could just get back to the bed then I could get comfortable and get back to my pattern of complete relaxation and be able to handle the contractions without a problem just like I had been doing before and like I had done with the previous two births. As I stood in the doorway, however, I felt like a complete wimp—what was wrong with me? I heard a feeble whine escape my lips. Then the contraction subsided and I got to the bed as quickly as I could.

Before I could get comfortable, another contraction came and then another. It came in to my mind what I needed to do at that point. "Listen to Kevin" is what the soft spoken voice in my mind said. Immediately I began to listen to him. He was telling me to breath. As I began to slowly release air from my mouth in a controlled manner, I began to realize what was happening. The baby was working his way down the birth canal now. Contraction after contraction kept coming with no break in between. I kept breathing out slowly, with some very gentle pushing. I could feel the baby coming down.

In the middle of this process, the midwife wanted to check the baby's heart tones again because she was a little concerned that his heart rate had been decelerating. I made some motion to signify that I needed to wait for just a minute. But the contractions kept coming. Pretty soon, the midwife figured out what was going on.

I had a very huge contraction in which, they tell me, my stomach shot way up into a point. I rolled over a little and crunched my body up somewhat during this. All of a sudden, the midwife saw the baby's head crowning. She gave a strong command for Kevin to get me flat on my back. As he did so, she quickly put her hand in under the baby's crowning head and pressed against my skin to help prevent tearing by such a fast birth. By the time Kevin looked over after the midwife's announcement of crowning, the baby's head was out. She was struggling to break the tough bag of waters. The baby's hand was flat up against his cheek inside the sack and there was meconium in the water. With another giant contraction, the rest of the baby slid out. Kevin was directed to grab towels and get this instrument and that. All this happened within about one minute.

The midwife told me just to relax while she checked the baby. He was perfect and beautiful and received a

10/10 on his APGAR score.  He was laid upon my chest as I lay there in complete amazement and relief.

From the time I was dilated to a five until the baby's birth was about 15 to 20 minutes.  That is incredibly fast! The midwife's assistant showed up shortly after the baby's birth.

As I look back on what happened, I believe that my concerns caused my labor not to progress in a regular fashion.  Once I cleared my mind of worrying about other things, that is when the contractions became regular and closer together.  Also, knowing that the midwife was a little concerned about the baby's heart rate, I think that at that point my body knew that the baby needed to get out pronto.  If he had stayed in me longer, he probably would have swallowed a bunch of the meconium water, which would have caused him problems.  As my midwife said, birth made it so that we didn't need to be concerned about his heart rate decelerating with contractions anymore.

Once again, there were miracles with birth. Heavenly Father had the best plan.  He knew what needed to happen.  Even right down to simply putting it in to my mind to concentrate on what Kevin was saying when the contractions started coming without any breaks.  I can not help but be amazed at how much heavenly help can be had during birth.

Of course I stayed awake pretty much all night because I couldn't possibly sleep while thinking of how very blessed I am. I lay awake and watched him sleep and kissed his little cheeks. Another precious baby to hold and love. Another little one that had come straight from the arms of God.

## Conclusion

As I said in the preface, every birth has the potential to be a great spiritually uplifting experience. I would not trade the miraculous heavenly interventions in any of my birth experiences for anything. It is when I have felt God's presence most abundantly. It is a most wondrous occasion.

Think of how Heavenly Father allowed His happiness to shine through at the birth of His Son – a new star, prophecies, multitudes of angels singing, peace, signs and wonders. While the birth of your baby won't be accompanied by such magnanimous wonders, you and your spouse will get a sense of the heavenly. After your precious bundle has arrived, proud papa may want to tell the world. Mama may look at her newborn and sense a peace and love there unsurpassed.

As you invite the spirit of the Lord to be with you in preparing for the miracle of the birth of your baby, may you be blessed to see miracles happen as you need them during your labor and delivery. May the power of God enhance your natural sense of wonder as you first embrace your newborn.

# ABOUT THE AUTHOR

Marika Lee Connole was born in Berlin, Germany to a Swedish mother and American father. She is fairly fluent in Swedish and has studied German as well.

Marika is the wife of Kevin Lee Connole and is a mother of seven children, most of whom she schools at home. She loves to cook, read and learn about things, would like to take up weaving again, and loves the challenge of creating something out of nothing.

She has a love of nutrition, having studied a lot over the years and having grown up working in a health food store. She wrote this book about childbirth hoping to help those who have not had wonderful experiences with birth. Marika has also written many homeschool articles.

Marika also enjoys music. She plays the piano, sings and composes music. She has the desire to work a little more on her limited knowledge of guitar. She also played clarinet once upon a time. Her compositions include everything from children's songs to ballads, to silly songs to upbeat medleys and hymn arrangements.

You can visit Kevin and Marika's website at www.completelee.com, to view all their latest products. Included on the website are many free items, such as, recipes, sheet music, coupons, games, articles and golf information. Contact Marika at birth@completelee.com. Share your story.